Florence Rosiello, PhD opened her private practice in New York City, in 1988. In 2008, she relocated her private practice to Sedona, Arizona.

Her first book, *Deepening Intimacy in Psychotherapy,* was published in 2000, Jason Aronson, Pub.

Dr. Rosiello is the Founder of Arizona Society for Psychoanalytic Psychology, and Arizona Psychoanalytic Society, Phoenix, Arizona.

To eight gay men.

Florence Rosiello

EIGHT FOUGHT TO LIVE

The Story of My AIDS
Therapy Group, 1988–1990

AUSTIN MACAULEY PUBLISHERS™
LONDON · CAMBRIDGE · NEW YORK · SHARJAH

Copyright © Florence Rosiello 2024

All rights reserved. No part of this publication may be reproduced, distributed, or transmitted in any form or by any means, including photocopying, recording, or other electronic or mechanical methods, without the prior written permission of the publisher, except in the case of brief quotations embodied in critical reviews and certain other non-commercial uses permitted by copyright law. For permission requests, write to the publisher.

Any person who commits any unauthorized act in relation to this publication may be liable to criminal prosecution and civil claims for damages.

All of the events in this memoir are true to the best of the author's memory. The views expressed in this memoir are solely those of the author.

Ordering Information
Quantity sales: Special discounts are available on quantity purchases by corporations, associations, and others. For details, contact the publisher at the address below.

Publisher's Cataloging-in-Publication data
Rosiello, Florence
Eight Fought to Live

ISBN 9781685628925 (Paperback)
ISBN 9781685628932 (Hardback)
ISBN 9781685628956 (ePub e-book)
ISBN 9781685628949 (Audiobook)

Library of Congress Control Number: 2023916935

www.austinmacauley.com/us

First Published 2024
Austin Macauley Publishers LLC
40 Wall Street, 33rd Floor, Suite 3302
New York, NY 10005
USA

mail-usa@austinmacauley.com
+1 (646) 5125767

To family and friends who
listened to each new chapter
and encouraged the next.

Table of Content

The Story of My AIDS Therapy Group: 1988–1990 — 11

Chapter 1: The Pink Cap — 13

Chapter 2: Long Eyelashes — 16

Chapter 3: Just a Quick Note About Group Process — 21

Chapter 4: Jason and His Argonauts — 22

Chapter 5: The Thomas' Crown Affair — 30

Chapter 6: Don't Come — 38

Chapter 7: Richard's Folding Chair — 41

Chapter 8: Just Once — 43

Chapter 9: Popcorn Ceilings — 49

Chapter 10: The Incident of the Easter Hat — 53

Chapter 11: The Kittyhawk — 57

Chapter 12: Mirrored Reflection — 65

Chapter 13: Needles and Threads — 71

Chapter 14: Tell Me Why — 77

Chapter 15: In the Beginning… — 83

Chapter 16: The Little Black Book — 91

Chapter 17: Guilt — 94

Chapter 18: The Socratic Method	96
Chapter 19: Thomas' Pain	99
Chapter 20: Down Mexico Way	106
Chapter 21: Cheerleading	113
Chapter 22: The Parent Trap	122
Chapter 23: Fabrications	127
Chapter 24: Waving Through a Window Dressing	130
Chapter 25: The Mink Coat	133
Chapter 26: St. Bartholomew	137
Chapter 27: Coda	140
Chapter 28: February 1990	145
Chapter 29: March 1990	151
Chapter 30: The Trouble with Taxis	155
Chapter 31: The Rain is Tess, The Fire's Jo, and They Call the Wind Mariah	157
Chapter 32: Getting Plastered	163
Chapter 33: Shoeless	169
Chapter 34: The House of Da-veed	173
Chapter 35: Raul	186
Chapter 36: Listening to the Unspoken	189
Chapter 37: Time	198
Chapter 38: A Promise to Not Die	200
Notes	**202**

The Story of My AIDS Therapy Group: 1988–1990

Chapter 1
The Pink Cap

These events are based on memory.

It was a private phantom and a pink one at that. Vito's pink cap looked like a yamaka with a brim. It wasn't an embroidered logo-allegiance baseball cap to the Mets or Yankees. It was just the kind of cap that makes your hair retain its shape long after it's been removed. This unencumbered and unfettered pink baseball-ish cap belonged to Vito Russo.[1] Only after he was gone, only after they were all gone, did the pink cap morph into an unattainable faint image darting in and out of my periphery.

"There it is," I always seemed to say that out loud, loudly. "Nope, gone again." My words seemed to slip out of my mouth and into people within earshot. There were other times when I just made sounds through an inhaled breath as though consuming a gasp, maybe a wish to absorb the pink cap inside me. Each pink glimpse reminded me of how powerful my anticipation felt, and every anticipation reminded my hope, to hope. Vito's pink cap just floated in the air, nothing or nobody wore it. It was my remembrance that engined this apparition. I owned this flying pink-fantasy for years and throughout that time, the moment it appeared, the next moment it vanished.

Just to be clear, I don't believe in phantom-y ghosts even though my childhood home was haunted by a female specter dressed in white that only my mother saw, but she'd had a few drinks, so who knows, and she'd only recently finished reading Wilkie Collins' book *The Woman in White.*

Still, it wasn't just Vito who colonized my inner world, it was all eight of them. Eight gay men with AIDS[2] who made up the therapy group I led at Gay Men's Health Crisis[3] (GMHC) in New York City.

At the time, GMHC was a new organization born in 1982 with the mission of helping and emotionally supporting gay men infected with AIDS, a rare form of cancer associated with malignant lesions, Kaposi Sarcoma. One supportive program GMHC provided was group therapy.

It was 1988. I was opening a private practice after having completed four years of psychoanalytic training, and I had it in mind to lead one such group. My rationale was that facilitating a group therapy would help build my practice, tone my clinical skills, and provide a referral source.

Soon thereafter, I arranged an interview at GMHC to lead a support group of gay men. During the interview I was informed that each group had around ten to fifteen members and two therapists per group. I guess two therapists meant a slower burnout rate. The following week, I interviewed the men who would make up this group.

Jason was a social worker who led AIDS groups for gay men at a local New York City hospital. Fernando was a published short story writer. Thomas an Oceanographer. Neil wrote poetry and was published. Chris was a Broadway theater actor/dancer/singer. Matthew worked as a window dresser at a large Fifth Avenue department store. Richard worked in finance in the Twin Towers. Vito was a published author, lecturer, documentarian, activist, and famous.

From 1988 to 1990, I shared the end of their life, and they unknowingly ended the life I led. Writing their stories has once again given them breath. My claim is memory of who they were and how they fought to live and lost.

This is my memory. This is their story.

Chapter 2
Long Eyelashes

I mustered up a bunch of narcissism as I was being interviewed by an administrator at GMHC during which I announced, "I'm going to run a group by myself because a co-therapist might not work clinically as I do, and I don't know what theoretical perspective they might adhere to, so I will lead the group by myself." Who knows what was up with this administrator or with GMHC because somebody gave the go ahead to lead the group solo when it wasn't their policy. The only thing I figured is the administrator wanted to teach me a lesson in humility or he thought having a psychoanalytic instead of a support group would have an interesting clinical outcome or because I told him I was going to write about the experience. Well, whomever this administrator was and who knows why, I got to lead the group by myself.

Sometimes we're instantly privy that something powerful is about to happen. In this case, privy meant jittery. As I was walking to GMHC for the first group session, I knew I was anxious, but I should have been a lot more anxious for a lot more reasons. Right off the bat, I walked past the building even though I'd just been there when I interviewed the eleven gay men who were to be my group. But now, on this very first day of our group session, each step seemed to stockpile apprehension. "I'm nervous," I thought out loud. To compound the situation as well as my anxiety, my out-loud talking was gaining volume. This broadcasted dialogue between mouth and mind preoccupied my feet and I walked and talked myself right past the GMHC building. To top it off, my internal conversation was becoming cranky.

"Why can't you remember which building?" One part chastised the other part. "Ease up," the other part reassured the chastised part. "Don't worry, lots of people in New York talk to themselves, out loud."

Eventually, both parts fell to defeat, "I give up. Go ahead, look like a tourist, ask for directions."

"Would you happen to know where GMHC is?"

"Up these two steps, lady."

"I need more navigational sophistication. At least fake sophistication," I lamented mumbling myself up the two steps.

"There's the receptionist." My palm tapped my head attempting to straighten thoughts.

"I'm here!" I announced to the receptionist who didn't share my surprise.

"Were they the wrong two steps?" I thought to myself out loud. I kept trying to stop my lips from inarticulate movements.

The receptionist was an adorable gay guy with the longest eyelashes. He seemed graceful and poised as he walked around the desk and gave me that come-with-me-hither look. As I moved toward him, he leaned into my hair and whispered, "I've been instructed to tell you there are only eight members now. Three died last week."

"What? I just interviewed them last week."

"They died since your interview." He leaned even closer to my hair, "Get used to it."

"Get used to it? Get used to shock?" I'm pretty sure he continued to talk as he led me to the group therapy room, but they seemed voiceless words. I was now walking on rubber legs that seemed to slingshot my knees together. My mind collided multiple thoughts into other multiple thoughts like Bumper Cars and bumped right out what Long Eyelashes was saying. "Is this my session room?" I asked right after he said, "This is your session room."

"Yes." His eyelashes met each other, maybe to keep me from seeing his eyes roll before he turned to leave. Alone in the hallway, inches from the door, not one piece of me could move. Instead, I desperately tried to negotiate with the three absent men, "Why couldn't you have waited?" My body was now totally stalled, until my stomach took the first step and sank into unknown territory. My second step mustered a slow smile as I turned and looked into the room. As Castaneda said, "In a world where death is the hunter…there is no time for regrets or doubts."[4] And so, I stepped through the doorway.

There they were, seated in a circle, waiting, all eight of them and three empty gray folding chairs. My initial anxiety melted into empathy as I slowly realized, "I will lose these eight men. I will lose all of them. One by one, they will disappear." In the next moment, my mind filled with despair, "Please, please don't think what I'm thinking."

I have no memory of crossing the threshold, but somehow I managed a feeble movement. Seeing them, my eyes couldn't stop battling my body's inner turmoil with the three empty chairs. Suddenly, chills ran every which way. "Which empty chair is mine?" A cacophony of rhetorical questions demolished any further movement. In growing panic, I desperately looked around the room wanting to shout, 'save me.' Save me? How ridiculous. Finally, one group member who seemed accustomed to hearing the unspoken, sensed the debate between my eyes, my body, and my decision. In a moment, he slowly leaned forward and without breaking eye contact, his face created a small smile arched in the direction of the seat next to his.

"Alright," I thought. "This is your moment. Go for it. Walk to his chosen chair." Nothing happened. Frustrated, I chided, "When did my mind and body all of a sudden become Cartesian?" Then, acrimoniously, "Oh, seriously, this is not the time to debate dualism." With that, I determined that my stalled predicament had nothing at all to do with me. I was not stuck. It was my shoe's fault. Yes, my shoes were the culprit. I glared at them, "Get going, move, now!" But seriously, we all know it's hard to move shoes stuck in hubris. Still, transferring blame to my shoes somehow quieted my internal criticisms and organized movement as I heard my shoe move the leather sole forward. Then, the other sole complied, but the sound of leather was quickly replaced by the click-click of my very high heels loudly greeting the concrete floor. I wanted to dissolve, but now Kafka started clanking around in my head, "From a certain point onward, there is no longer any turning back. That is the point that must be reached."[5] I'd reached it.

Finally, I came face to face with the chair next to his. As I turned to sit, the chill from the cold metal folding chair acknowledged the shallow depression in the back of my knees. With a relieved sigh, I glanced at my shoes, now gratefully thanking them for not betraying me. My face humbled a smile as it lowered my body to the chair. I straightened my Laura Ashley dress, reminded my smile to stay put, then looked around at the remaining men and announced, "Let's begin by introducing ourselves."

"Shouldn't we wait until the others get here?"

"They won't be coming," I uttered into dead silence. I've often wondered how music critics are able to describe emotional effects of listening to melodies and sounds because the dirge of 'they won't be coming,' was a repeating chorus in my head.

The chair next to me breathed deeply and in a swelling whisper avowed, "No one else dies in this group." We all froze in attention. Again, he repeated it, but now louder and as a demand. "No one else dies in this group." The power and deep intonation of his voice meant to claim blood brothers. Eight bodies shifted as though movement was promise to not die.

Chapter 3
Just a Quick Note About Group Process

Every individual in a group, in a group therapy or even in a family group, well, everybody negotiates with everybody to find their place, their role so to speak in the group's development and functionality. Some individuals become more powerful than others, others emotionally distance themselves, a few feel lucky to be included, one or two get scapegoated, and some just buck the group system altogether. These developments can be smooth and seamless or feel like a casting call audition for a Saint Vitus[6] dance troupe.

Typically, it takes a few weeks before group members realize their self-relegated role. However, when Jason issued his decree 'no one else in the group dies,' there was no joust, no jockeying, no negotiation. Jason took the lead right smack dab in the first session and throughout the entire life of the group he held the coveted role. He became the voice of and for the group. For the next two years, no group members challenged nor competed for his position, and I would have been alright with that, except it was my role.

Chapter 4
Jason and His Argonauts

In Greek mythology, Jason, the rightful king must prove his birthright to his uncle Pelias, who stole the throne from Jason's father, King of Lolcos. As a result, King Pelias sends Jason on a mission to find the Golden Fleece; a symbol of authority and kingship because Pelias wants Jason out of town. To aid in this journey, Jason enlists the most important heroes of Greece who become known as Argonauts, named after their ship, the Argonautica.

There was one female hero who was also entitled to be on the Argonautica. Her name was Atalanta. Unfortunately, women were not really wanted as an equal on a ship. As a result, Jason left Atalanta behind, agreeing with the Argonauts that a woman should not belong in a group of heroic men, even though the ship was built by a female, the Goddess Athena.[7] You get the metaphor, right?

Sitting next to Jason in this first session, I could feel his intensity. Probably because his folding chair rocked a little bit when he spoke. After his pronouncement, I found myself watching him, indiscreetly of course, from the corner of my left eye. Then, within a split second my periphery magnified as Jason made an exaggerated, almost courtly turn in the direction of my left ear. My chin folded to my neck, as my head backed up for a safer viewing position to squint left at him. He smiled at my squint and just like a kid who finished licking the frosting off the cake-mixer whisk, he surveyed the seven other men in the room. To be more specific, his facial movement took on a planet observatory spin, scanning everybody's face. Then with intent, his hand tapped his knee and without a care in the world or even any desire to share the cake icing with anyone in the group, he pitched, "So, who wants to go first?" Silence. "Great!" Without waiting to hear an answer, Jason joyfully proclaimed, "Alright, then I'll go first." He hesitated, apparently remembering group etiquette, then sang out, "Oh, of course, if it's alright with you all, I'll go first." The self-chosen leader looked absolutely delighted while the rest of us felt a little taken aback or maybe it was just me, probably.

The group hummed with variations of agreement or maybe it was relief of not going first. I could have hummed, too, but I was still a little stuck in my head. Adding insult to injury, my taken aback part seemed to have gotten smothered in muteness. Yes, that was it. Jason muted me.

With his self-created entitlement, Jason began leading *my* group. He must have decided I was in no shape to start the group, especially since I had trouble walking from the door to my chair. Maybe so, but my mind was loudly protesting in my indignant moment, "It's me who's supposed to start the group session." I didn't say out loud. During this in-my-self-moment, the professional part of me dwindled into an absolute justified lamentation about being demoted. My offended and silenced-self protested, "Hey, you know, I'm the leader here. I'm supposed to go first." Then in full-fledged growing resentment, I scolded my clinical training. "Why didn't anyone teach this in therapy school, i.e., how to work with Jason-dynamics in an AIDS therapy group." This was exactly the same feeling of invisibleness I used to feel in Kindergarten when I wasn't picked by the 'good' team to play Relievo. "Pick me! Pick me!" Here I am, still stamping my feet just like when I was five. However, since Kindergarten I learned invisible people often have trouble in the real world, which is probably why I announced, 'I will lead this AIDS group by myself' to the GMHC administrator. So, I resorted to my Kindergarten technique and tried to seem cavalier and not care one hoot about being overlooked while the others played without me.

"Who does Jason think he is?" I insisted to myself whilst struggling to grow up and return to adulthood and some smidgen of professionality. "They're leaving me/Atalanta behind. Isn't this an age-old story," I ruminated. Jason had taken the helm and the AIDS group/Argonauts were on board. It was as though he shouted, "*Everyman*[8] board ship! We set sail at first light!" Then he says, "Oh, yeah, Atalanta (that's me), I know you're an *Everywoman* hero, but, you know, you're not a man." Now, I have to tell you whenever I get on a literary roll it's hard to rein back even during a first AIDS group session. I sat there, on that hard gray folding chair, silently chastising Jason for wanting the golden fleece. In another snarky second, I thought, "Well, first he has to find that gold furry thing and while he's doing that, I can go to the administrator at GMHC and tell him to give me the fleece and return my role to group leader." I shook my head in reprimand, "Maybe I don't really need a fleece. Jason can keep it. Just for this session."

Returning, who knows how to the real world, I heard Jason assert, "I have a Master's Degree in Social Work and I'm an AIDS group leader at the AIDS Hospital up the street." Right. He *actually* has his own ship, and I am *definitely* Atalanta. I know there are other things men have that women don't, but that's not the point of what I'm trying to convey here. So, to recount, Jason had more clinical, actual hands-on experience leading groups of gay men with AIDS way more than I did. The only experience I had was happening right now and I was in my own way.

In hindsight, during the life of the group I never lost foreboding of becoming Atalanta. Was I necessary in this group? Here I am invited to board the Argon, but noooo, I have to be content and hang by the pier and watch the men get, fleece? It's interesting how dramatic foreshadowing isn't evident until it's over and that's why I don't like dramatic foreshadowing.

"Maybe having a co-leader is a good idea, as long as it's not me who's the co-leader," I mused trying to convince myself. "Co-leading could lessen the stress of leadership." Then, within yet another second thought, I devolved right into paranoia, "Did GMHC sneak Jason in as co-leader?" Luckily, there was an unspoken policy that mental health workers who lead groups at GMHC should not have the AIDS virus, so I was safe on that front. This unspoken policy/rationalization is that a leader who had AIDS might visually deteriorated (or die) and if so, it might quicken the demise of other group members. I think this was it.

Jason was still commanding the ship when my mind returned to the group's discussion and heard various voices challenging Jason.

"Isn't that an AIDS overdose?"

"Why?"

"You lead an AIDS group and come here to *be in* an AIDS group?"

"That's incredible!"

"Aren't you on disability?"

"No. I'm good."

Let's face it, who knows better to lead an AIDS group than someone with AIDS. Cat was out of the bag, and I heard myself snarky muse, "GMHC thinks otherwise." On the other hand, maybe Jason's co-leading was some GMHC administrator on a white horse trying to save me from solo group leading. Finally, I found my voice somewhere and with a pretty smile, "I want you to know, I'm very glad to be here." Then, conjuring up a tad of professionality, "I enjoyed meeting you all during the interview. I think you guys will be a great group, a good group."

"Did you interview some people who you didn't think would fit in?"

"Some, yes. For various reasons, some people were better for other groups." A few of the guys smiled, some nodded and Jason didn't do either. I've always wondered if Jason saved my seat because of that *The Godfather* movie quote, 'Keep your friends close, but keep your enemies closer.' Paranoia has a way of feeding on itself and mine was a little hungry that day.

Just to be clear, Jason wasn't really an Argonaut. Actually, he looked like Clint Eastwood in *Rawhide,* albeit

Clint with a mustache. Jason had those long slim dimples that took up most of the lower part of his face and deepened when he doled out a smile. As time passed, I learned he was serious, stoic, sarcastic and, I admit, special.

Jason had a full head of beautiful hair, just like Clint's *Rawhide* TV hair. I remember worrying, "I'm not supposed to be thinking this much about Jason. I have a group of men here and this Clint Eastwood wringer shouldn't be distracting me." At other moments, I silently retaliated my self-reprimands with, "Nothing's wrong with Clint thinking." On the other hand, I really needed to calm down.

"Why *Rawhide*?" Then it occurred to me, while I was walking to GMHC, I'd passed a gay bar, aptly named *Rawhide*. It was a bar for gay guys 'into leather.' By the late 1970s, there were a lot of people, straights, and gays, who were into rawhide leather bars. I mostly knew this because I lived in an apartment down the hall from two of the sweetest gay guys who ever graced leather. Every so often, if I was coming home late, they'd be all dressed up in chaps, jackets, vests, motorcycle caps like James Dean in *Rebel Without a Cause*, or was it Marlon in *The Wild Ones*, or maybe it was Travolta in *Grease*. It probably was *Grease,* but more probably it was Olivia Newton-John's leather outfit because it really made an impression on me. Anyway, my down-the-hall neighbors went to the leather bars in the Meatpacking District of Manhattan, not far from GMHC. I am not making up any of this.

It was one of my gay neighbor guys who became an early AIDS victim in 1978/1979. After he died, his lover of twenty years was evicted, even though they'd both lived in the apartment that amount of time. The rumor was the landlord didn't want to rent to someone with 'the gay disease.' This soon became the saga/norm in NYC apartment rentals. Honestly, my neighbor, the one who survived his lover, he died a year later from AIDS, but I think there were broken-heart complications.

Jason reminded me of these neighbors because he could have that tender oxymoron-leather-look, as well. He could have been a Hollywood heartbreaker film-star with his just-right-tight-jeans and top three shirt-buttons, unbuttoned. He had a smooth, muscular, hairless chest that if you sat in exactly the right spot next to his folding chair and if you stretched your neck a little bit you definitely got a better view of those buttons.

Jason had deep brown squinty eyes that peeked out of his Clint Eastwood face and sad bedroom eyes. Sometimes sitting close as we did, I wished I could experience his emotions for him, providing a break from his own intensity. But intensity is inherent in an AIDS group and merging, taking on the patient's feelings as one's own, flew in the face of my just-finished psychoanalytic certification. Merging was definitely not a good clinical idea.

During analytic training, one of the theories we learned proposed that therapists are participant observers, not participants. But here, working with these men, being an observer felt too impassive and disconnected. As time passed, I began to reconsider the analytic theory I was adhering to, Self Psychology. It just felt too emotionally distant for the men in my group. Here they are, dealing with life and death and I'm being distant? I had to change my clinical approach, which is no easy feat. It's like saying, 'I need to build a new house.' Be that as it may, I had to be more emotionally related, more real, and more focused on deepening relationships and intimacy with and between these men. Luckily, in the 1980s, a new theory was developing. It was labeled Relational Psychoanalysis, and the emotionality inherent in this theory fit the bill entirely. The men in my group needed to feel my emotional presence, my caring, and my respect for them. If they are being real, I'd better *get* real.

Seriously, look at them, young, attractive, articulate, funny, a bunch of genuine individuals who every day feel the awfulness of living with AIDS. But, what are these feelings? What is the emotional level-of-intensity that exists in waiting to die? Before I began leading this group, I included myself as someone who 'understood' many types of emotions. But I didn't, and still don't. Then and now, I will never have a clue about living with AIDS in the late 80s, early 90s.

I remember the group discussions about not having a full life, about the public not caring or doing anything about AIDS because it was 'a gay disease.' During these sessions, I often felt furiously overwhelmed that they/my men would die. I wanted to yell out and demand an answer, "Who infected you? Who gave you AIDS? Who did this to you?" Early on in our meetings, my mind's inquisition painfully pressed, "Why aren't *they* wondering who gave them AIDS? Why don't *they* confront whomever it was that infected them?" Then, it hit me, reality penetrated my incensed interrogation. If they knew who infected them, they might also know who they infected.

Chapter 5
The Thomas' Crown Affair

It was probably the following week I decided that since I was the *real* group leader, I didn't need to struggle with Jason for the role. Let's face it, we were both aware of our place at GMHC and our place in the group. If Jason needed to feel in control and powerful in the group, then well, shouldn't he have power over some part of his eclipsed life? It also made sense the other members would identify with him because they had the same need. Some people might interpret that I chose a passive position, but I seriously doubt my friends would ever describe me as passive, then or now. Rather, I felt it was important to provide these men with some sense of control and authority somewhere in their lives. In hindsight, I still agree with myself back then.

On this Wednesday evening, a week later, I was absolutely delighted at my ability to walk across the room without reprimanding my shoes or needing Jason to tell me where to sit or struggle over who begins the session. Jason could be quite pleasant and gentle when not challenged. "Let's get more acquainted tonight. You go first," Jason's command was directed toward the tall blond guy, Thomas. "Sure, I'll go first." Thomas glanced at me for confirmation.

I nodded and he began, or maybe Thomas was looking at Jason who was right smack dab next to me. The tall, blond man's voice held a solemn, resigned tone, "My name is Thomas and I've had AIDS for almost four years." He shifted in his chair, perhaps gathering himself or his pride and announced, "I'm an Oceanographer." He quickly held up a finger indicating pause for correction. "I mean I *was* an Oceanographer, now I'm on disability. To be absolutely correct, I'm a disabled Oceanographer with AIDS on disability." He scanned the group, then sardonically, "Don't you think it's ironic that AIDS and disability are bedfellows?"

I must admit, Jason's choosing Thomas was a good idea. Still, I *still* had moments of recurring bouts of envy. Narcissism can be powerfully pompous.

Thomas was in his mid-forties. His physical presentation was striking. There was a regal quality about him that complimented his six-foot stature and perfect posture. His hair was strawberry blond hair, and he wore very cool-looking aviator glasses that matched the color of his hair. I thought the shape of his glasses made his eyes look a lot sadder, though.

Listening to Thomas, he seemed to speed-read/blow off his archived oceanic credentials as if he was taking a high school history test with Mr. Hughes, who never passed anyone, so why care about significant details.

The more Thomas spoke, his articulation, intonations, and his New England accent really sent my imagination lickety-split. I had images of King Charles the First, generously bestowing Thomas' aristocratic royal ancestors a huge chunk of land in the New World.

I shook my head to untangle fantasy from reality and forced my attention on the real Thomas. His hand movements, his smile, and his crystal-clear sea-blue eyes were magnetic. His voice was silky and mirrored the smoothness of his transparent porcelain skin. It was as though you could see, or maybe 'sea' through his skin right into his heart.

Thomas' posture was perfect. He sat absolutely straight, as if he had gone to military school. Which led me to ask, "Where are you from?"

"Massachusetts," Thomas proudly responded.

"You lived there most of your early life before coming to New York?"

"Yes, I lived in Massachusetts until I came to New York to work."

"Did you go to school there or here?"

"Do you mean college or high school?" Thomas queried.

"Both, why don't you start from the beginning."

Suddenly, I realized Jason was staring right into my left ear. He looked appalled. I'd forgotten he was supposed to be group leader. My job was to keep the folding chair warm.

At the time, I was pleased with my questions to Thomas. In hindsight, they were a little robotic and I should have given Thomas time to elaborate. I'd also ignored Jason's desire to feel important. But I was just out of analytic training and did what I thought I'd been trained to do. So, I sat back and congratulated myself. I was done for the remainder of the evening, and I let Jason take over, again.

"I went to Tabor Academy," Thomas responded, genially.

"Where's Tabor?" A new voice chimed in, "Oh, I'm Matthew. Sorry to butt in. I've heard of it, but don't know where it is. I'm from Massachusetts, too."

Smiling as welcomed introduction, "Marion, Plymouth County by the ocean." Thomas looked away, perhaps musing his next sentence. "Actually, it's called the School by the Sea. My father wanted me to go there, and I shocked him by agreeing. That's about all we ever agreed on."

"After Tabor, I went to the Courant Institute of Mathematical Sciences at New York University. My internship was at Woods Hole Oceanographic Institution. I got my doctorate at Princeton in Atmospheric and Oceanic Sciences. After all that, I worked as a marine conservation scientist until I switched to disability."

"Did you take classes in Mermaid? I'm Neil, by the way."

"Yes. I got extra credit for having the biggest tail."

Everyone was smiling, laughing, "Good for you," announced the curly red-hair guy. "I'm Chris."

Encouraged, Thomas continued, "Unhappily, my big tail landed me here tonight."

"What got you interested in oceanography?" Matthew's voice was gently inquisitive.

"My father was an oceanographer," Thomas responded with absolutely no hubris whatsoever. "My grandfather was an explorer, a seaman, as was my grandfather's father and on and on." Thomas inhaled deeply, "Actually one of my ancestors was a *Speedwell* pilot; the ship that was supposed to accompany the *Mayflower*. I've been told that during one of its many voyages, an ancestor of mine piloted it. I don't know if that's where the family fascination originated. Who knows, maybe we were Vikings."

"That threw me for a minute, Thomas. Oh, I'm Richard. When I think about pilots, I think about planes not ships," Richard chuckled, making his folding chair tip a bit.

"Thomas, that's an amazing story," someone chimed in.

Jason interrupted, "Remind us of your name." Jason was on it, doing the job he wasn't hired to do.

"Oh. I'm Fernando."

Thomas nodded, his voice returning to the curriculum vita, "To finish up, I deal with partial differential equations, turbulence, fluid dynamics, chaos theory, statistical mechanics, data mining. Stuff like that."

"Right. Now we know exactly what you're talking about except I don't know what you're talking about," Fernando shook his head gently mocking Thomas' eruditeness.

"I can't begin to imagine what it feels like to follow in your ancestors' footsteps. You're talking about centuries. For centuries your family has explored the ocean. That is impressive. I'm Vito, by the way."

"Vito, as though you need introduction. There's nobody here who doesn't know you," Chris laughed, his red curls flipping punctuation.

Apologetically, Vito asserted, "Thomas, could you continue? Sorry I cut in."

"Yeah, I want to hear more about this, too." Richard's folding chair rocked a bit when he spoke, "I'm impressed. How often do people follow their father's, grandfathers, and lots of great-great grandfathers' careers that go back to, well, to the beginning of time? No, I'm curious. What kind of pressure did you go through to keep the oceanographer line going?"

Thomas hesitated, "You guys really want more of this?"

Jason interjected, "Absolutely. We need to talk about ourselves otherwise what good are we to each other if we don't know each other."

"As detailed as you can get, is great," Vito spliced into the discussion.

Thomas heaved a sigh, "Well, yes, I followed a long line of oceanographers but as far as my father was concerned being gay erased my achievements. Pretty much erased me," he chided. "In my father's mind, being gay and being his son was an absurdity." Thomas exhaled, probably in exasperation. "Honestly, his need for me to be straight was rough on everyone in the family, but my being gay was nothing compared to the maelstrom when I told him I had AIDS. I thought he would never recover."

Thomas looked right at me as though wanting to avoid a more emotional discussion, or perhaps a request for permission to tell more. On second thought, he was probably looking at Jason. "Finally, my dad gave me a look that could kill and with all the disgust he could conjure up he laid it out, 'Well, Thomas, you certainly got what you deserved. If you got AIDS, that's your problem.' Then, I heard him say under his breath, 'It's her fault. The way your mother over-protected you. She made you gay.'"

Thomas scowled, "My father is such a hypocrite. We found out a while ago, he's been having an affair for the last twenty years." Thomas' voice became mockingly sing-song, "But, did my mother leave him when she found out? No." Emotion mounting, "My father bullied and lied, and guilted her about how she'd be abandoning her children if she left him. My sister and I were adults, for god's sake. A couple days later, I heard him tell my mother that she couldn't leave him because no one would love her the way he did. What crap!" Thomas stared at the floor as though his father's face was in the concrete, and he wanted to step on it. "She bought it. He's such a bully. Anyway, like I said, he hit the roof when I told him I've contracted AIDS. Later, my mother told me try to be more understanding because the news of my having AIDS was embarrassing for my father." Thomas threw his hands in the air in exasperation, "Okay, I'm done. That's enough for now."

"Why? You're on a roll. Keep going."

"Nah, I'm done."

"Seriously," Matthew interrupted. "Someone else's story might be worse than yours, so keep going."

Jason crashed his hands like symbols, "Come on, we want to hear."

In that moment, Thomas' frustration became a cornerstone for an emotional brick wall, anger brick on anger brick. "Alright, here goes. My father was like a damn drill sergeant when we were kids. Whenever I was home on holiday breaks, I had to sit next to him at dinner because I was the oldest. If ever I put my elbows on the table, he'd swat them with a spoon, right on the bone to make sure I got the message. His spoon smacks made bruises because he hit so hard." Thomas smirked, "Now, I make sure my elbows are always on the table every holiday meal and I sit far away from him. But that doesn't stop him, he says, 'I paid all that money to send you to a good school and they didn't teach you how to eat like a human being?'" Then, oozing sarcasm as though speaking to his father's image on the concrete floor, "Hey Dad, I put my elbows on the table. I have sex with men. I got infected just to piss you off."

Everyone was silent, maybe waiting for Thomas' father to vanish. "I'm glad you told us about yourself," Neil consoled. The group was buzzing, commenting on Thomas' story, offering to tell their experiences in upcoming sessions. They offered empathy, sympathy, and camaraderie. While I watched their excitement, an undertone of insignificance came over me. These group members held purpose for each other, a promise to each other, a vow to live, to have a future. My purpose in the group, well so far, I didn't really know, but I knew I had to 'get used to it.'

Chapter 6
Don't Come

After a few weeks, crossing the threshold into these newly created weekly-sessions offered relief. No empty chairs. In addition, I felt the group was slowly accepting me or perhaps Jason loosened his grip on the throne realizing I was not plotting a coup. Probably both. Even so, I've never stopped wondering if the GMHC administration guy was nuts in letting me lead solo.

It was during one of these early-on sessions that Jason told me what was expected of me as 'group leader,' which is somewhat paradoxical, but at least he acknowledged I *had* a role in the group. "It's important for you to know protocol regarding our hospitalizations, because we *will* be hospitalized."

"Okay," I responded cautiously.

He was looking right into my eyes, "If you go to the hospital every time one of us gets sick, you won't make it for very long. You'll burn out and be useless to the group." I was surprised. Jason was saying, 'You/me might be useful.' So, I accepted the unspoken compliment. Let's face it, Jason obviously knew what was in store for an AIDS group leader.

Jason cleared his throat, then loudly announced, "When we get hospitalized, we visit each other, we show up. We go. Not you. You don't go." His statement emotionally engulfed me like a mist slowly forming a specter of the future. Of course, I knew at some point they would go to the hospital, but I didn't want anyone to say that out loud. Out loud made it even more real.

Surveying everyone's face, it was clear they agreed with him. Honestly, I knew Jason was right. I did know about some therapists at GMHC who visited their group members in the hospital, and they did burn out. Some of these therapists emotionally fell apart. That's a better way to put it.

Without looking up, no, I'll be honest again, without being able to look up, I reluctantly agreed, "I will not visit any of you in the hospital, but I do wish that wasn't so." They were right. Of course, they were right, but being right doesn't keep wrong wishes from replacing right ones. Still, wouldn't they be just as burned out if they went to each other's hospitalization? Wouldn't they be overwhelmed at repeatedly seeing the harbinger of their own future?

Jason kept right on talking, or maybe lecturing is a better way to put it. "One more thing we need to discuss and it's probably something you won't like because it's not in the rule books."

"What?"

"I know people in group therapy are not to socialize outside sessions for a variety of therapeutic reasons. For one thing, you (he meant me) are not privy to how we're relating to each other. The reason this rule exists is because relationships that develop outside our meetings can get complicated and there's no way for you to know what's happened or to ward it off. But we need every bit of support we can get. It's important we have access to each other because we keep losing people who used to be our support. Do you agree to our meeting socially outside the group environment?" Was this a question?

"Well, socializing outside the consulting room is not an accepted option for members of group therapies for a variety of reasons, as you mentioned Jason. It has the potential to form clicks or to create issues that should be discussed in the group sessions. In addition, you're right, it also excludes the therapist from group dynamics that can alter or terminate the direction of the group process."

I didn't say any of that. What I blurted out was, "Absolutely, you should meet outside." What else could I say? Should I have said, "I know you guys have lost friends and lovers and, well, that doesn't matter because according to group therapy technique, I am expected to restrict the friendships you might create with each other outside group sessions. It also doesn't matter that those group therapy boundaries were established long before any AIDS group was formed. These group therapy rules still apply." I didn't say any of that, either. I'm not going to say that to men who desperately need each other and who won't be around in a couple of years. "Yes," I smiled ear to ear. "Absolutely! Absolutely! You should meet outside group sessions."

"That's great." Jason confirmed that I'd just said the best thing possible.

Chapter 7
Richard's Folding Chair

Richard was a little different from the others in our group. He got along with everyone but at times he could be a beat behind on social cues. Interestingly, he had no idea he was late. Richard believed he was good at reading social cues and not only was he good, he was correct. From his perspective everyone else was a beat behind. My assumption is that Richard never read Heidegger because Richard's subjectivity only included Richard's perspective.

In our sessions, when Richard wanted to be acknowledged you'd better snap to it. Here's the Richard/Likert Scale of Attention: First, he'd lean forward, then slide himself to the very edge of his chair. Next, he'd sit ramrod straight like Punxsutawney Phil, so you just couldn't miss him. If that failed, he'd very slightly bop around on the chair. All that to say, it was sort of amazing to watch Richard because it was reminiscent of Joe Cocker at Woodstock in '69.

Richard, just a little, reminded me of Ernest. The kid I sat behind in third grade. This was way back in Trucksville Elementary School which is now an old age home and the irony of that is weird. Anyway, just like Richard, Earnest had stages/levels of getting attention if he wanted Miss Trimble to call on him. I remember once Miss Trimble asked a question directed at someone sitting on the other side of the room. Earnest wanted to answer but he was on the wrong side of the room. So, he raised his arm and started waving his hand a little bit, then a little bit more until finally I got worried all the blood was going to drain into his armpit.

I was also getting upset about Miss Trimble's eyesight. She didn't even see him when everybody else could sure see him. Somebody had to do something, so I stood up and started pointed my fingers toward Ernest trying to match my finger pointing with the cadence of his hand waves. To my surprise, it only took about a second for Miss Trimble to notice. Back then, I was stumped as to why she told *me* to quiet down.

All that to say, Richard could get your attention. I'm positive Earnest was not related to Richard.

Chapter 8
Just Once

Richard worked on Wall Street until about a year ago when the stock market plunged on 'Black Monday.' He hoped when the market recovered, he'd find another financial position. A few group members still had jobs. Still-having-a-job was interpreted as potential for longer life. Unfortunately, I worried the market recovery might last longer than Richard.

I remember this one particular session where Richard was very intent on getting everyone's attention, "Listen, I would like to talk about my lover." Richard took the 'Punxsutawney Phil' position, so we did notice him. "It's the anniversary of our breakup a few years ago. I can't begin to explain how emotional it was." Richard sat back, then leaned forward, "We both worked on the Street (Wall Street), so we had a lot in common and tons to talk about. Frank and I, well, we first met by coincidence. I'd seen him around, but nothing more than that. One evening after work, I decided to join co-workers for a drink. I don't drink much, but lots of people go out for a drink after work. Let me clarify, lots of Wall Street people really *need* a drink after work. I thought if I went along, I might be able to talk to this cute guy, Frank. I wanted to get to know him. Like I said, I don't hardly ever drink so I'd ask the bartender to make my ginger ale look like it was a Margarita. After a few weeks of seeing each other at the bar, Frank and I drifted to a private table, away from co-workers. We both just seemed absolutely drawn to a small, secluded table so when the crowd thinned out, we'd sit at 'our table.' The more we saw each other at the bar, the more intimately we talked, and eventually, more lovingly. It was so yummy being with him." I remember getting stuck in my thinking when Richard said he felt 'yummy.' However, Richard might eventually provide yummy definitions, so I remained in listening mode.

Richard's face beamed, "I used to love looking into his eyes and feel his caring. Under no circumstance did I want to rush the relationship and told him I didn't want to sleep with him before we really knew each other. I remember Frank looked at me, sort of surprised when I said that. At the time, I figured Frank must not have had many people be so open with him. I wanted him to really know me, so I told him all about my life."

"You enlightened him?" Fernando joked, but Richard didn't hear him.

"After about six months I figured we'd dated enough, established a good connection, and now it was time for sex. As luck would have it, one evening we both got a little drunk."

"I thought you had ginger ale," Matthew interjected.

"Usually, but this one evening they gave me a few 'not virgin' Margaritas by mistake and I was slightly looped, which, thank goodness, gave me the courage to invite him to my apartment."

Jason sarcastically responded, "Right. Of course, Richard, we've all had a spiked virgin Margarita."

"Ha, ha, Jason. Very funny," Richard laughingly sneered.

"Oh, I'm sorry, Richard. I couldn't resist," Jason said apologetically. "I do want to hear about what happened with Frank."

"Thank you." Richard continued, "As I said, both Frank and I had too much to drink, and believe me Frank drinks way more than I do. Even so, there was no way he could take the ferry to Hoboken."

"So, I said to him, 'Stay with me tonight.' I told him I would probably need help getting into my apartment. I said that even though I knew he wanted to come home with me."

The longer Richard spoke, the more his face took on a faraway quality, as though he was emotionally reliving this experience. "My apartment is beautiful. It overlooks the Hudson, and you can see the ferry going back and forth to Hoboken and Frank said he was glad he wasn't on it. He said he'd missed the last ferry of the evening, so he felt okay staying at my place. I knew what he really meant. He wanted to stay and make love to me. We had another drink and he pretty much held on to the walls getting to my bed."

At this point in Richard's story, he seemed to be dangling precipitously into another dimension. "I undressed him. I knew Frank wanted that. Then, I slowly undressed myself, so he could watch. He was so coy, he pretended he was asleep. I was really, really nervous and not sure I could even do it because I'd had way too much to drink, but I didn't fail, and Frank rose to the occasion."

Richard's voice softened, "I stroked his body in such a loving way and I could hear he was breathing heavily, so that meant he was ready. I was gentle. I knew him well enough to know he wanted me to take charge. He wasn't a virgin, I knew that. He talked about other guys he'd met at bars and had sex and never saw them again. He frequently went to the t-room (toilet room) at the Monster Bar in Sheraton Square, and he was no stranger to the meat market bars." Was Richard bragging about Frank's conquests?

"Frank said he had sex in so many t-rooms, he lost count of how many. Probably over a hundred. I knew he was really meaning I was different because he actually knew me. It felt so tender, you know what I mean?" Some group members nodded, but Richard seemed oblivious.

Richard's facial expressions began to morph into a hypnogogic trance; that dreamy state philosopher Thomas De Quincy wrote about in *Confessions of an English Opium Eater*. De Quincy boasted that opium use created 'a phantasmagoria of dreams,'[9] an extended opportunity to live within fantasy and Richard looked like he was slipping into De Quincy's reverie. "That night was magical." Richard sighed dreamily, "I held Frank in my arms all night long. He looked beautiful. Our lovemaking was beyond surreal." Richard closed his eyes, perhaps trying to intensify the image of their lovemaking or symbolically performing 'blinded by love.'

"The next evening after work I went to meet Frank at the bar, but he never showed up. I waited and waited." Shaking his head, Richard lamented, "I went to his office the next morning. Both of us worked in the Twin Towers. Frank in the North and my office was in the South tower. I went to his office, and he wasn't there. That's what his secretary said. I thought it was strange because I could see Frank's jacket hanging in his office. Then, I thought he probably just forgot his coat."

Richard opened his eyes, "All of a sudden, it hit me, he probably needed time to think about the intensity of our incredible relationship last night." Richard sighed, "I called his office a couple times just to check on him. His secretary was a little huffy and told me he was really busy, and he'd call me." Sighing relief, "Then, I knew for sure Frank was overwhelmed by the potential future we would have together. He just needed time to adjust."

Richard's mood began to alter, as though consoling his world and his words. "After a week, I couldn't take it anymore and went to Frank's house in Hoboken." Suddenly, Richard gushed in excitement, "Oh, it was a really, really nice house. A big house. It took him forever to get to the door, but he eventually invited me in, and I sank into a beautiful plush light blue damask davenport. Frank sat on an oriental cherry-wood chair with lots of mother-of-pearl inlay. He asked if I wanted coffee and I said 'sure.' He served it in a beautiful art deco silver coffee set." Richard still seemed entranced. "I was so excited. I thought, 'Oh, I like everything he likes.' It was incredible. I started daydreaming about the wonderful life we could have together living in this house." Richard's imagery continued, "While Frank and I were drinking coffee in his beautiful home, I brought up how fantastic our sex was that toasty night we spent together. Frank laughed; he'd had too much to drink and said he didn't remember much. I kept talking, very sweetly, trying to jog his memory. Frank was listening but becoming fidgety, probably embarrassed his memory was foggy." Almost with bravado Richard recounted, "Knowing him as well as I did for the last six months, I changed the subject to protect him from more embarrassment, so I asked him, 'How was work?' 'I've been slammed and, oh, I have news,' Frank declared. 'For the last few weeks, I've been seeing someone. You'll meet him when he comes back from the store.'"

Richard's face fell. His voice barely audible, "I felt crushed, but I kept remembering he was probably just blown away by emotions, probably trying to run from the powerful love we made together. Frank just couldn't love this other man the way he loved me." Richard's voice tightened, "Our night of pure desire, the sexual intimacy was frightening him. Of course it was. I felt so sad on the Ferry ride back to Manhattan, poor Frank caught between two lovers." Richard's voice softened to a whispered, "That was the last time, and that was the *first* time I ever had sex. I know the exact moment." Richard's voice cracked in agony, "I know and I love the man who infected me."

Not one of us spoke; not one of us moved. Richard's confession was deafening. His words kept reverberating in my head, as if Quasimodo was in the belltower repeatedly ringing, 'The first and only time I had sex.'

Richard's confession seared itself into my conscious mind. While we all heard it, only I have remained to live with it.

Chapter 9
Popcorn Ceilings

As time passed, I entered GMHC each Wednesday evening fully aware my men would be in the session room way before me. This was their time together, time to joke with each other and probably tell stories deemed unfit for the female group leader. These conversations usually dwindled when I entered the room.

It reminded me of high school when the teacher was late for class. We'd be throwing number two pencils in the air to see who could lodge it into a popcorn-ceiling crevice. Sometimes we switched from pencils to spit balls. The trick was to create the most desired, the largest spitball-worthy-of-an-award-sized spitball and catapult it onto the blackboard. We were a group of teenagers pledging unity, an action, a behavior that made us feel powerful against the teacher's authority and control over us.

This was similar to the growing unity among gay men with AIDS. They united against the media, the FDA, the drug companies, and then forced the government/the authorities to recognize their power as a group.

Gay activism created easier access to medications and lowering the cost of AIDS drugs. In 1988, in just one year, there were roughly 10,911 *reported* deaths from AIDS in the United States. Between 1981 and 1988, the cumulative total was 46,134 deaths.[10] This group of statistics also wield power. It was when the popcorn ceiling pencils surrendered to gravity, or when the spitballs dried up leaving their mark on the black board; it was then our teacher knew we had power to disrupt and re-direct her attention. It was when gay men with AIDS became activists, when they showed the power of unity, they received attention, felt empowered, and believed they could alter the future. When the eight gay men in my group came together, their bodies were weak, but together they too felt a powerful unity.

I could hear them chattering as far away as the first-floor stairwell. As I got closer it was easier to decipher whose voice was telling a story not predetermined for me. On this evening it was Vito. I never interviewed Vito. He was a gift from a GMHC administrator who announced Vito would be in my group and only attend sporadically 'per his lecture schedule.' "It'll be great to have him in our group. Thank you." I knew Vito was author of *The Celluloid Closet* because I'd read it, and that was the extent of it. The administrator did not say anything about Vito's AIDS activism nor about his involvement with ACT UP (AIDS Coalition to Unleash Power).[11] He didn't tell me Vito lectured throughout the U.S. as well as internationally on gay rights. He didn't say Vito lectured at a California university where he taught classes on gays in film. He didn't mention that Vito wrote, produced, and co-hosted a local television series entitled *Our Time* on public television. You know where I'm coming from on this, right? Embarrassed. Totally embarrassed. As a result, I just pretended to know everything about Vito. Pretending is a good thing. It's incredibly creative.

Vito probably had the most exciting, stimulating, and glamorous experiences of anyone in the room. When he told a story, it was excellent. Sometimes he'd talk about an ACT UP rally, how he felt standing at the podium giving speeches to thousands of people, or he talked about the famous people he knew, Lily Tomlin, Liz Taylor, Madonna, and many others.

On this evening, I delayed a tad more before entering the room to eavesdrop because, well, because I wanted to know ahead of time if the number two pencils were going to fall from the ceiling. In addition, I knew if I walked in, Vito would politely wrap up his narrative, lean back on his folding chair and become *just* a group member, just one of the guys. But let's face it when you're special, you can't become un-special.

After successfully eavesdropping, yes, it was probably a little longer than necessary, I walked in. Maybe my manner was slightly strange/guilty because they immediately shifted their discussion and stared at me. "What? What? What are you looking at?"

"Your dress. We're looking at your dress." Much to my chagrin, they started riffing.

"What? It's just my usual Laura Ashley dress. Alright, yes, it's new." I was funnily indignant.

"No," Matthew teased. "This dress is different. Turn around so we can see it."

"No, absolutely not." After some mutual back and forth, they won, and I did some Vanna White *Wheel of Fortune* movements in the middle of the folding chairs. When I finished Vanna, I sashayed to my chair next to Jason. Looking around, I knew I was still in trouble and so held my breath waiting for the spitballs to fall off the blackboard.

Neil cleared his throat, then mockingly, yet politely asked, "Do you have a dry cleaner's garment conveyor in your closet?"

"Not a large one." I was going with the flow. I tried to mimic Vanna White's voice even though I never heard her speak, but whatever. "It's just a small conveyor."

"Ten to one, you've got the entire second floor of Saks Fifth Avenue in your closet," Matthew chimed in.

I protested, "Isn't that the children's clothing department?"

Matthew taunted, "You know very well the second floor is the designer department."

Thomas joined in, "Well, I know her dress didn't come from the peppy clothes on the third floor. The pink and green stuff."

My Laura Ashley dress was mortified. "I don't wear pink and green stuff," I huffed double-checking my dress.

Richard waved to Thomas, "How do you know preppy is on the third floor?"

"Seriously? If anyone knows preppy, I know preppy. You're looking at the king of prep."

Everyone was joking and laughing, and I didn't care if I was the initial recipient, odd man out. These eight men were united, and I was totally alright with number two pencils lodged in the popcorn ceiling.

Chapter 10
The Incident of the Easter Hat

It was February 1989 and I decided to beat the crowd and make a quick detour to Macy's to buy an Easter hat. Easter hats still sold like hot cakes, and I really needed one. Luckily, I found a yellowish hat with a millinery daisy on one side, and a cute short veil that was fashionable back in the 1980s, which meant my hat wasn't fashionable very long. While I succeeded in beating the Easter hat crowd at Macy's, there was a problem I didn't anticipate. If you buy a hat, the store puts it in a hatbox. Hatboxes were big, round, hard cardboard cumbersome box things, hard to maneuver on the subway or on a windy street, or through the hallways of GMHC. I wanted to get to the group before any of the guys so I could hide it. I was concerned the size of my hatbox might symbolize the size of my narcissism, and both felt embarrassing at the time.

As luck would have it, I was wearing my very trendy blue swing coat hosted by enormous 1980's shoulder pads capable of sheltering three or four short people standing in the rain at the bus top. The plan was to hide the hatbox under this blue gargantuan swing coat so nobody could see it. "Ah, empty room. I'm here first!" I said twice, sounding like a frightened five-year old. I tucked my coat around the box, making sure the folds looked casual thus promoting the notion that nothing was under my coat other than a big, round hump in the middle. "Perfect, no one is going to see you," I said to the hatbox, as though reprimand would frighten it to stay hidden.

As an aside and at that time, if I'd had more experience as a therapist, I would have known everything has potential to distract therapy from therapy, and it is the analysis of distractions that enhance opportunities to understand the unconscious. Meaning, I just should have let them see the hatbox.

Turning my back to the hat, I heard the guys chatting as they walked toward the group room. I shot a stern look at the hatbox as an additional warning to keep it together. The guys entered the room in the way many people get onto subway cars, trial and error.

They were probably surprised I was already there, probably more surprised my coat looked pregnant. By now, they knew I sucked when it came to having a poker face. They all seemed to mull over the visual/mental process of 'she's early and her coat is pregnant' and just like slow motion instant replay they stopped in their tracks.

"I knew it," I said out loud in my head. "What?" I actually said out loud.

Neil squinted, "You've got the my-dog-ate-homework look." Still in slow motion or maybe I entered some fugue state, they smiled and gave me that jig-is-up smirk. Chris broke free from the stalled group members and began to move toward me. I could see his red curls flicking fire sparks, indication I was in for it. Then, he turned and stared at my pregnant coat. It was a wonder to watch Chris' red hair magnetically detecting the location of my hat. I don't remember if it was Zarathustra or Nietzsche who wrote about time, movement, spin, and pursuit, but it sure explained Chris and his hair in that moving moment.[12]

My hat was no longer an innocent bystander. It took on portions of its own and morphed into Sirens luring Ulysses/Chris over the blue water/blue swing coat as he parted the coat from the box. There it was. The hatbox, fleece, whatever. With great aplomb, Chris opened the box and dramatically removed the yellow hat with the cute little veil and held it like a laurel wreath as though he would crown himself. Lo and behold, Chris slowly placed the hat on his head, tilted it with a pop from his hand, walked into the center of the folding chairs, and we all knew to take our seats. The show was about to begin.

Chris leaned back, then slowly slid one foot forward as he pushed his shoulders blades back as far as possible. He was listening to music we were only just beginning to 'hear.' Then he stopped, looked up, looked down, ran his thumb and finger over the brim of the hat, and stepped sideways as we disappeared into his mind's audience, fifth row center. His gold top hat sparkled under the spotlight as he moved to well-known choreography from *A Chorus Line* and began singing, "One singular sensation…"[13]

Fifth row center came back into view, and we all jumped up to provide a standing ovation. Chris bowed while we shouted, "Bravo! Bravo." In the next moment, the room resounded with variations of, "How do you know all that?"

"Where did you learn the choreography?"

"That was incredible!"

Kudos floated through the air filling the room with excitement.

Chris smiled, "I was in *A Chorus Line*." He took a deep breath, then lowered his eyes as though closed eyelids meant the curtain was down. He spun around then plopped onto his folding chair. A moment later, without looking up, he leaned forward offering me the gold top hat. It took a long time before I reached for it. I was in no hurry to take back my yellow hat with a daisy.

Vito whispered something sounding like, "…the stars."

"What'd you say?" Neil muttered back.

"It's a line from a movie," Vito responded, almost inaudibly.

"What? We didn't hear what you said."

"Oh." Vito conceded, "Don't let's ask for the moon, when we have *the star*."[14]

Chapter 11
The Kittyhawk

"I have some good news. I know good news is novel in these times," Neil announced, his face glowing. "Another one of my poems was published."

"I didn't know you wrote poetry," Fernando blurted out. "How come you never mentioned it? You know I write. You never once mentioned it."

"Oh, geez, it's just poetry. That's different than writing a whole book. It's nothing more than poems," Neil humbly uttered.

Matthew interjected, "I'm impressed that anyone could even *write* poetry, much less get it published."

Chris seemed awestruck. "I'm impressed that I actually *know* a poet."

"Getting anything published is quite a feat," Fernando chimed in.

"When did you start this? I mean when did you start writing poetry?" Chris' excitement was charming.

"I started in elementary school. I mean, nothing happened to those poems except they're in a box in the back of my mother's closet. But, in high school I wrote the poetry column in the school newsletter. I guess that was like a publication, except I was the editor and that made it easy to get the poems printed. You know, it wasn't until college, until one of my professors encouraged me to take poetry more seriously, that I took it seriously. I had some poems printed in *The Tufts Observer*."

"You went to Tufts?" Thomas exclaimed.

"I did."

"Where's that?" Chris interrupted.

"Massachusetts."

Thomas perked up, "Tufts! whoa! Wait a minute, didn't Tufts just have a disciplinary issue? It made the papers, didn't it? Yeah, it did. I remember reading it."

"I know. It made the papers." The cadence of Neil's voice became cautious.

"Yeah. That was some incident." Thomas slid to the end of his chair, inviting more discussion.

Neil vigorously shook his head in confirmation, "Yeah, I didn't know the guy. Some of my friends did, though."

Thomas nodded, "Well, Tufts is a liberal university, so I was really surprised that incident happened. Even more so, that it got published in *The Associated Press*."

Jason interrupted, "What incident? What are you guys talking about?"

"Good question." Chris conferred, then urged, "Yeah, what story?"

"Neil probably knows more than I do." Thomas was eager to hear the inside scoop.

"No, actually. I don't know much more. Thomas, why don't you tell them what happened."

Thomas acquiesced, "Sure. The story I read in *The Associated Press* said a student wrote an article condemning racism, this was at Tuffs, and it was published in the university's newsletter. *The Associated Press* picked it up after the guy who wrote the article was beaten up by a couple of guys." Thomas slid back in his chair. "It was just last year, maybe a little more than a year ago when I read it."

Neil confirmed, "I think so. The guy got beaten up badly. Which is probably why it made the papers."

"Is he alive?" Chris interrupted.

"Yeah," Thomas and Neil responded in unison.

"But he *really* got beaten up. He was hospitalized," Neil added.

Matthew was intrigued, "What happened to the guys who did that?"

"Well," Neil sighed. "There were people who saw it, but they denied it was an attack. They said nothing really happened." Neil shook his head in disbelief.

Thomas jumped in, "If nothing happened, why did the school settle the case out of court? Why did the story make it to *The Associated Press*?"

"Was the guy gay? Was that why he was beaten up?" Richard interjected.

"Yeah. Was he gay?" Fernando echoed.

Jason oozing sarcasm, "He was gay, I'd bet. He was probably gay. Was he?" Everyone in the group was full-on interested.

Neil shook his head, "I don't know. I have no idea, but who knows. I know the guys who beat him were white."

"We all know just being gay is enough reason to beat him up, you know," Jason sarcastically interjected.

Thomas' eyebrows became incredibly tight. "Strange because Tufts is an exclusive school. They don't like scandals. It's a sophisticated university, so you'd think they wouldn't have students who would have done that." Thomas shook his head, "It's hard to get accepted into Tufts. How did they let thugs into Tufts? You went to Tufts. You said you used to live in Massachusetts."

Neil smiled, "I went to Tufts, but I grew up in California. My folks were born in California. My father was from San Diego. My mother grew up in Sacramento. My father was in the Navy. They met at a dance, a Navy dance."

"That's romantic," Matthew cooed.

"Yeah. He was in the Naval Air Force in the early 1960s."

Intrigued, Richard asked, "Did he fly a lot?"

"He was one of the Air Force pilots on the largest aircraft carrier in the Navy, the *Kittyhawk*." Neil looked uncomfortable, "Are you sure, you want to hear this stuff?"

"Of course, we do!" Chris announced.

"Alright." Neil looked around, "Do you guys know about the *Kittyhawk*? The first aircraft carrier?"

"Oh, sure," Thomas nodded.

Neil hesitated, "I'm conflicted about telling this." He inhaled deeply, "Never mind, I may as well talk about it. You've been telling your background. I guess it's my turn." He cleared his throat, then cleared it again.

"Yeah," Jason retorted smiling. "We want to hear it. We aren't going home until we hear it."

"Alright. When my father was around twenty-two, he was a Lieutenant in the Naval Air Force. He wanted to fly since he was a kid. My mother said he wanted to buy his own plane after the Navy. I don't remember how he got assigned to the *Kittyhawk*, but somehow, he did." Neil stopped, then double-checked everyone's face. Perhaps still apprehensive about revealing more.

"Like I said," Jason jokingly threatened. "Nobody leaves until you tell us what happened."

Matthew chided, "I have absolutely no intention of sleeping on folding chairs tonight, Neil, so, let's hear it. You grow up around the Navy and your father lands planes. What's the rest?"

Neil leaned forward, "No. On second thought, you guys don't want to hear this."

"Of course, we do!" Chris exclaimed.

"Neil," I interjected. "Are you worried we'll get upset or are you worried about remembering what happened?"

"I *do* want to talk about it, but there's no happy ending here."

"Well, that's something we're never faced with," Jason retorted sarcastically. Then added, "Go ahead Neil, we can take it." You had to give Jason credit; his sarcasm was ever ready.

Neil forced a weak smile, "Okay, so the *Kittyhawk* is an aircraft carrier, and my dad flew one of the planes on the ship. My dad was a pilot in a three-man plane. Well, let me go back a little bit." Neil inhaled, gathering air to swell his story or maybe to get strength to tell it. "Landing planes on a landing path, on a ship, isn't easy and back then, they were still perfecting how to land and take off. You're doing both from a moving ship. A ship on all kinds of waves."

He continued, "According to my mother, my father was lead pilot in a three-pilot plane and it was his job to land it on the ship." Neil shifted in his chair. "This one time when he was landing, he came in too low and the plane hit the ship's deck. One of the wings cracked or maybe it broke off. I think the wing broke off. I'm not positive." Neil cleared his throat, "When something like that happens, you've really got to react fast. Which he did. My dad reacted so fast, he managed to get the plane back up. It's a big deal to get the plane back up into the air, especially with a cracked wing." We were all mesmerized by Neil's story. "Somehow, my dad got the plane up high enough that the crew, the other two pilots had enough time to bail out." Neil's shoulders sank.

"This really is hard for you to talk about, Neil," Chris comforted.

Neil shook his head, "No, no, I've told this much. I'll tell the rest." Again, he inhaled deeply, "When you bail out of a plane, you must follow rules of 'reverse rank,' which would be seaman first, co-pilot next, and lead pilot last. My dad was lead pilot." Neil's voice tightened, "It took a lot of skill to land those planes on the *Kittyhawk*. Somehow, my dad gets the plane back up high enough for the seaman to jump out, and for the co-pilot to jump out. These two guys ejected incredibly fast and fell right into the ocean. They were rescued by the guys on the ship." Neil cleared his throat, "My mom said, my dad couldn't eject. There wasn't enough time." Neil's words quickened, "The damaged wing hit the water and when a plane hits water, it sinks. The hatch won't open under pressure of water. There's no way to eject from a plane that's sinking. You can't eject with water above you." Neil inhaled, "I was born two weeks before he went down. I never met him." For a few sad moments, I think we all held our breath.

"You never met your father?" Chris said tenderly.

"No. Never did."

Neil tried to smile. "When I die, I'm going to be buried next to his headstone. It's just the headstone, there was no body because he went down inside the plane. My mother and I have been looking at headstones, so I can have one like his."

"What! You're looking at headstones?" Thank God nobody said that.

After a few moments, Neil scanned everyone's face. "Way back in the past, people in my family used to have a poem engraved on their headstone." His voice fell to a whisper, "I might be a poet, but I haven't been able to write a poem for my own headstone. There's no poem on my dad's headstone, yet." Neil paused. "Wait a minute." Neil leaned back, reached into his back pocket, opened his wallet, and pulled out a worn piece of paper. "Here's what I've come up with. I don't know who wrote this, well, nobody does, it's anonymous. It works for what I want for my dad. I feel like it works for me and my father. Do you want me to read it? I don't have to read it."

Jason reacted quickly, "Yes! Read it."

"Are you sure?"

"Yes," Chris looked around gathering confirmation, "Am I right, guys?" Everyone agreed.

"This is what I'm thinking should be on his headstone. It's not the whole poem, I'll just read the last couple of lines."

*"Do not stand by my grave and cry,
I am not there,
I did not die."*
– Anonymous

Neil's mood surrounded us. Struggling to continue, his voice cracked, "If you've never met your father, then in your mind, in my mind anyway, if you've never met him, he's never dead. He was just who I wanted him to be, who I wished him to be. When I was a kid, I decided that my father is who I want him to be and I'm who he wanted me to be."

I heard Thomas mutter, "Not in my family. I'm not what my father wanted, and he's not what I wanted." Neil didn't hear that. I'm pretty sure he didn't hear.

Chapter 12
Mirrored Reflection

"Let's start the group." Of course, Jason announced that before I said, "Let's start the group."

Vito quickly interrupted, laughing, "I got to tell you, this group is inseparable." There he was, smiling under his pink cap. "I just hung out with all of you two days ago." Vito turned in my direction, "We all went to the movies!"

In a split second, Chris started singing the old walking-popcorn-box advertisement from the 1950s, 'Let's all go to the movies.' An aside: Actually, it was 'Let's all go to the *lobby*.' You were already at the movie. It was time to buy more popcorn and another box of 'Good & Plenty.' I didn't say any of that. Instead, smiling like a proud parent, I agreed, "You guys are definitely close. So, what'd you see?"

Neil chuckled, "What else, the *Dead Poets Society*."

Fernando added, "It was excellent!"

"Yes," Vito broke in. "Of course, there is an undertone of two characters being gay. One of them wants to be an actor, to the chagrin of his straight-as-hell father. Well, in the film, the son suicides and the audience is left to assume, this is from my perspective, the son suicides after his father rejects him for beings gay."

"There it is!" Thomas slouched on the hard-gray folding chair, obviously frustrated with his personal struggle of straight father/gay son.

Returning to Vito: During all the time I led the group, I never met anyone who wasn't enchanted by Vito. If you knew him, you almost automatically respected his brilliance, intellect, humor, and mannerisms. Maybe there are people out there who didn't admire him but it's probably just one or two. I felt lucky he was in my group. We all did.

It wasn't until the group's formation that I learned about Vito's lover, Jeffery who died in '86. Jeffery's death and Vito's mortality harmonized his vulnerability with his activism. Vito's stories were often naked to the bone, laced with outrage or peppered with tenderness. For instance, his speech at the ACT UP Demonstration in Washington, DC on October 10, 1988.

An excerpt from Vito's speech at that rally. *"...you know, living with AIDS in this country is like living in the twilight zone. Living with AIDS is like living through a war which is happening only for those people who happen to be in the trenches. Every time a shell explodes, you look around and you discover that you've lost more of your friends, but nobody else notices. It isn't happening to them. They're walking the streets as though we weren't living through some sort of nightmare. And only you can hear the screams of the people who are dying and their cries for help. No one else seems to be noticing."*[15]

Vito was right. There was stonewalling from drug companies and misrepresentation from the media about the gay plague. This discrimination rang louder for Vito and his activist colleagues. Relentless individuals like Vito Russo organized and band together confronting injustice and deceit from the drug/medical community about AIDS and AZT. Vito was fighting for change and a chance to live longer.

It was during this session, I began to notice Vito's skin tone. It looked different today. He was more pale than usual, and his skin had gray undertones. The space above his upper lip seemed sunken, as though skin met bone without muscle. These symptoms were signs of increasing illness. I glanced at the others in the group. Surely, they saw this, too. Vito's symptoms were slowly impacting the emotional texture of the group. We were all getting quieter. What was going through his mind? What images were falling to the cutting room floor.

"You know," Vito lamented. "Today when I was getting ready to come here, I was talking to my mother on the phone while I was shaving." His voice wavered, "My mother and I were chatting about usual stuff, you know, family stuff. Before we hung up, she said, 'I love you.'"

"I love you, too, Mom." Vito scanned everyone's face. "I do love my mother. I love all my family." He hesitated, "My mother's love, my family's love, it's just not like Jeffery's love. It's not like what Jeffery [Sevcik] and I felt for each other." Vito smiled, perhaps floating to memory. "Yet, we were, well, some of you know, we were almost totally opposite personalities." Vito's shrunken lips struggled to maintain a gentle grin. "Of course, there were things we didn't agree on. I liked being out there, I mean loudly out there, in the thick of things, being an activist and

Jeffery didn't. It wasn't for him." Vito tone stumbled, "He'd just go into himself. We didn't want to change each other, we just wanted to be who we were, who we had been, who we could have been, together."

Vito smiled again, a faraway smile, "I mean, don't get me wrong, sometimes I did things Jeffery told me to not do, insisted I not do, like when I told him I was coming to San Francisco. He was dying." Vito's voice pitched, "I *had* to go there to take care of him. I *wanted* to take care of him. Jeffery was so sick. He did *not* want me to come, but I didn't care. I went. Of course, I went." Vito sighed deeply. "He was difficult toward the end. Unmanageable, I mean. He was physically and emotionally deteriorating. I wanted to keep taking care of him, but over time, he was running me down. It became so stressful." Vito's face altered; he looked tortured. "I wasn't with him when he died. I was on a flight from Melbourne to Honolulu. No matter what I did, I couldn't get a seat on the plane from Honolulu to San Francisco. I had to wait an entire day before flying out. Jeffery died that night. He died when I was in Honolulu." Vito's voice cracked, "I wasn't there. I wasn't with him." Vito shook his head until the pink cap faltered in the wrong direction.

"I miss him. I miss our love."

He paused, "I was thinking about Jeffery when my mother and I hung up, after she said, 'I love you.' I finished shaving but for some reason I kept looking at my reflection. I told the mirror, 'I am going to die with no one loving me the way Jeffery did.'"

I was stunned, everyone was. I slid to the edge of my chair ready to blurt out, "What are you talking about? We love you!" Luckily, I was speechless. It was obvious Vito was mourning a lost future within intimate romantic love. Our platonic love, the group's love was not the topic. Vito made a statement of what he felt. No one's opinion has bearing on what someone else feels. I said nothing. No one spoke. I've always wondered how did we *all* know to remain quiet?

In these seconds of silence, Vito adjusted and lowered the brim of his pink cap, perhaps wishing to hide or block view of us. Either way, everyone sensed his needed privacy. On the other hand, maybe we all needed solitude because when I glanced around, no one was looking at anyone. Richard was slumped in his chair. Matthew rolled his sleeves up and rolled them down. Jason angrily stared at the floor. Chris folded his arms and joined Jason in floor staring. Thomas looked lost. I stared too, because I saw everyone else staring.

Looking at Vito wasn't an option because who wants to stare at someone in mourning. The easiest averted eye movement in that moment was onto my lap. Within a few minutes and without awareness, my fingers somehow intertwined and took refuge on my flowery Laura Ashley dress. Deep red roses, blue cornflowers, honeysuckle, lilacs, lilies of the valley, all bouquet together guiding a memory into the garden of my dress. These flowers look just like the ones I saw in a park in Norway.[16] Rows and rows and rows of roses. Huge rose beds wide awake, all leading to an enormous monolith of sculpted humanity. It was a beautiful totem. Romanesque sculpted bodies, intertwined, each dependent, all resting on the curled stone-body above and below." My daydreamed relief faded, interrupted by the sound of Jason shifting his folding chair, bringing me back to the session. No monolith. Just my dress. Why now was my conscious illuminating this memory of body resting on body? Why have I signed up to watch men die?

Chapter 13
Needles and Threads

The following Wednesday evening session began almost immediately after I sat down and even before Jason could begin the session. Vito cleared his throat, his eyes enormously wide open. "Listen," he cleared his throat again. "I have just been informally informed that our documentary on the quilt, *Common Threads*, has been nominated for the next Oscars." [17] An immediate loud 'whoop' resounded the room, excitedly followed by accolades of, "You're kidding!" "Wow!" "Amazing!" Some of the guys jumped out of their seats in excitement to applaud, others hooted and hollered. They were so loud the folding chairs rattled like nobody's business. Everyone talking over everyone, "Oh my god, Vito. When? When are the Oscars?"

"March, next year (1990) in LA. Billy Crystal is hosting."

"Unbelievable!"

"He's fantastic!"

"Oh, everyone will watch the Oscars if Billy Crystal is doing it and the quilt documentary chinches the deal."

"Everyone will watch!" Vito's smile was so wide you could see every single tooth.

"We're just nominated, you guys. We haven't won, yet."

"Are you kidding!" Chris yelled, red curls flickering.

"It'll win an Oscar, and I'm coming with you to see it!" Chris looked in my direction, "You've all seen it, right?"

I totally knew that question was meant for me and not Jason.

"Yes!" I lightly bounded once on my chair in keeping with the group's mood, "I've seen the documentary. This is so fantastic!"

Vito nodded with enormous enthusiasm, "I can't tell you how wonderful it feels. I talk about Jeffery in the film. Of course, he'd probably hate being made so public." Vito's face softened, "They show the quilt at the end of the documentary. It's powerful! If you haven't been to DC to see it, you should go."

Richard interjected, "Of course we've been to DC!"

Thomas smiled, "No, I haven't seen it yet. I will, though. I plan to see it." In the next moment, Thomas' chair felt far away. He was still sitting there, but somehow became emotionally absent. Finally, he muttered, "The quilt." It almost sounded as though Thomas' inner world spoke. 'The broken threads of yesterday, the deserted seat, the closed book, the unfinished...'[18] Thomas sighed, "The unfinished quilt."

Fernando whispered, "What'd you say?"

"It's from a Dickens story," Thomas mumbled.

"Which one?"

Thomas smiled, "It's one of his short stories, *The Haunted House*."

As the mood relaxed, the conversation eventually morphed into 'requirements for adding patches to the quilt,' which quickly led to 'how many have patches have been sewn together,' to 'what's the most recent count of how many deaths from AIDS.'

It wasn't all that often that Vito's schedule allowed him to attend sessions, so the moment the conversation lulled, and because he was an integral part of ACT UP, I asked, "Vito, what's happening with ACT UP? What's the FDA status on AIDS meds? I've read the newspapers on this, but they're biased. Could you catch me up to date?"

"Of course. Sure. Well, you know what we've done so far. The activism, I mean, right?"

"To a degree. I know about Wall Street, I mean the Stock Exchange protest. I've heard about the protests against the drug companies, in particular Burroughs Wellcome. I know about the Sloan-Kettering four-day long protest."

"That was a good one," Neil interjected. "So was the protest that closed down the FDA."

"Yeah, they arrested almost two hundred of us," Neil responded proudly. He chuckled, "That was one crowded jail, for sure."

Jason questioned my left ear, "What else do you know?" Without waiting for my response, he asked, "Did anyone tell you about Vito's speech. The speech he made at the Albany and DC rallies?"

"No," I responded plaintively. "I guess you guys were there and heard it."

Thomas lamented, "Yeah, I couldn't make it, though."

Chris' curls chimed in, "It was fantastic! Riveting! Tell her about it, Vito."

"No, that's okay."

"No, it's not okay," I gently argued. "Could you at least tell me a little about what you said?"

Vito, hesitated, then, "Sure. Essentially what I wrote is, 'One day when this AIDS crisis is over, when people finally know and realize that, well, that a group of very brave individuals decided to fight by protesting, everywhere and anywhere we could to get the straight world's attention and to get them to help us."

Vito smiled, as though pleased to do Chris a favor. "So, we protested," Vito continued. "'If we don't protest, others might not live and be free from this disease.' That's pretty much what I said."

In the next moment, Vito's smile faded. "We have a lot of doctors helping us, but they're overwhelmed just trying to keep so many of us alive. Do they even have time to care for those of us who are infected but not dying? Plus, they're fighting all kinds of political stonewalling and fighting drug companies who are getting fat off our deaths." Vito's frustration was elevating, "This is one of the problems. Doctors are fighting the same thing we're fighting, the drug companies, the politics of the FDA. The drug companies are deliberately holding up medications that we need now, not later. We need them now, so we can stay alive." Vito's agitation climaxed, "We have to get organized. I mean the doctors and the protesters need to talk to each other and strategize. We have to consolidate efforts so we can kick the shit out of this disease." He paused, took a deep breath, then looked at all of us. "We need to kick the shit out of the system, so this never happens again." Vito exhaled, "That's pretty much what I said at the rally." [19]

Jason moved to the edge of his seat, leaned forward, and began clapping. Neil joined, then Matthew, Richard, Fernando, Chris, Thomas, all methodically clapping the way the French do after a concert. Chris jumped up providing a standing ovation, his curls happily accompanied him. Richard followed suit, always ready to shake up his folding chair. The room felt wonderfully alive with hope for the future, and anger for the present.

"Oh. There's one more thing." Chris leaned forward, "You guys, I want to tell her what else happened at the rally. I can't believe none of us mentioned this before. Did anyone tell her about the DC rally?" A rhetorical question, apparently because Chris launched right into the story. "We're at the Washington DC protest. All of a sudden, there were a whole bunch of teenagers driving around, and they started heckling us. Not a big deal. We ignored them. I think they were drunk. Apparently, they didn't want to be ignored. They stopped their car and started yelling, calling us names, mocking us. So, one of our guys at the rally turned on his boom box." Chris shot me a look, "Yes, gays carry boom boxes, too. Well, in the middle of everything, to drown out the crap the teenagers were yelling, this guy at the rally gets up and starts playing loud disco music. Then, a bunch of us got up and started dancing. It was contagious because then everybody around us started dancing. We drowned out the noise the jerky teenagers were making and just kept dancing."

Chris shrugged and smiled ear to ear, "It didn't take long for the teenagers to give up and go away." Somehow, his red curls slowed down, "Oh yeah, I heard somebody say something about 'with all the horrible things going on, with all our deaths, look who we are, how we join together, how we made something bad become something good. It's amazing what we're able to do together. Here we are, at a rally in DC, united."

Why do they have to rally, to fight to get medication? Why isn't it just available? Why does one pill cost $8,000.00? I became lost in silent indignation.

"It's late. Let's wind up."

Everyone nodded.

"Yes, it's time," Jason added.

"See you next week." I waited until they were gone, until their voices diminished down the hall. After a few minutes, I put on my large blue swing coat and walked to the door. Then, I remembered to double-check if anyone forgot something. I spun around, looked back into the empty room. Eight empty chairs. How in the world am I going to get through this?

Chapter 14
Tell Me Why

About a month or so later, maybe mid-way through the session, Jason leaned in my direction and out of the blue, at least to me, loudly asked, "Hey, I want to know, how come you decided to run this group? Why do you want to be here? You don't have AIDS and you're not gay. Why are you here?" Then, more emphatically, "What's in this for you?"

"Think fast," I told myself, which at 9:00 on a Wednesday night isn't my forte. "Well, originally I figured this experience would help hone my therapeutic clinical skills." I didn't say that. Nor did I say, "to provide a patient referral source." These two original motivations were now embarrassing, naive and sounded as if I was using them. What should I say to Jason? I mean, since being connected to GMHC, my private practice *was* booming. Gay men referred gay men. Gay men referred lesbians. Lesbians referred lesbians who referred a ton of lesbians. For a straight lady, a straight female therapist, I was now considered an LGBT-friendly therapist. I can't say that to Jason and I felt humiliated my practice was doing well.

There he was again, talking to my left ear, "Why are you still here? Why are you still with us?" I glanced at him, then stared at the floor. Maybe the floor could cave in and I'd be swallowed up. My thoughts felt like desperate inmates struggling to escape. Suddenly, my unconscious released memories. It was like being rabbit punched. This was the very first time the real reason came into my awareness.

"Many of my friends, two of whom were special friends, died from AIDS. They passed so quickly they didn't have time to tell me they were sick." I shook my head, then fell to sadness. "Our mutual friends told me they were dead. I was shocked." Then I mumbled, "You know, I can't seem to get used to being shocked."

Jason interrupted, "That's why you came initially. Why do you keep coming here? Week after week, why are you still coming?"

I swallowed hard. "There's no one reason. Perhaps in part, because being here, listening to you has made me see and experience the emotional intimacies of life very differently. What I feel each week is a juxtaposition of admiration and fear. Why would I leave life's importance? Everyone in this group, well, you all seem to have prioritized time and relationships. When I started here, I thought I knew how to be a therapist. Just say the right things, ask about feelings, use interpretations sparingly, and focus entirely on the patient. I didn't realize I was part of the mix, nor did I realize the importance of my vulnerability." I inhaled quickly. Actually, I was probably hyperventilating.

"In the beginning of our group, I thought theory was crucial the clinical process, but the theory I was using back then, when we started, just didn't work in here. If I was going to be *with* this group, I had to be *in* this group." I looked at their faces, "You want more? No, you don't want more, right?"

Jason pounced, "Yes, *I* want more."

In that moment, I wished my mouth had a mind of its own because I had no idea of what else to say. Then I thought, where is Jason going with this? I'm being manipulated. "You know Jason, sometimes people ask a question when they really want to answer it themselves. Why are you asking?"

Before he could respond, Thomas' baritone intruded, "Jason, I'm curious too. What's up?"

Neil interjected, "Why do you want to know why she returns each week? You've been running AIDS groups every day at the hospital."

"It's different, I have the virus," Jason's body shifted on his folding chair.

"I hope I answered your question, Jason."

He took a deep breath, "Listen, I've had a bad day. Let's drop it. Forget what I said, forget the question, the topic. Over and out."

"You're kidding. This is group therapy. We don't drop anything, we don't quit a topic, and we don't quit being here," Neil countered.

Matthew went right to the point, "Jason, why do you run AIDS groups at the hospital? There are other social work jobs."

"It gives me a reason to drink at night," Jason retorted.

"Well, you don't have to work in a hospital to do that," Neil said sarcastically.

Within a split second, Richard's chair squeaked from movement, "This is a little different from Jason's question."

He was looking at me, "I've wondered what's it like when you leave here after group?"

"Seriously?" I whined.

"Yes, seriously," Richard was adamant.

"Well, after group I get in a taxi, and on the way home I watch people on the sidewalk, especially people walking around Chelsea, because so many gays live in Chelsea. Sometimes I feel scared and start to worry. How many gay men on this street are infected? How many have AIDS? How many can't get help? Then, when I finally get home, I over-tip the driver because I'm totally preoccupied with ruminations." I paused, to organize more thoughts. "When I leave here, I usually think about the session. I feel overwhelmingly sad that the only thing I have done for you guys is create this group. It's frustrating because you give so much to each other. You socialize, especially around activism. I can't chain myself to the banister of the Stock Exchange, or lie in the aisle of St. Pat's, go to rallies, or ACT Up meetings. I can't do any of that. I see patients all day, some who have AIDS. There's no extra time for protesting or activism, and you guys wouldn't approve of my attending, anyway." Sitting straighter, "So, Richard, when I leave here, I think about each one of you and I feel frustrated *this* is the only thing I give you."

Thomas gently interrupted, "Speaking for myself, I don't need you at the Stock Exchange or at St. Pat's. We have enough activists, we need caregivers."

Jason snapped back, "I'm a caregiver *and* I protest with ACT UP."

"Jason, what's up? What's going on?" Neil looked angrily concerned.

"I'm just upset." Then, seemingly unable to contain emotions, Jason blurted out, "Actually, I don't do both. I just got let go from the hospital. They eliminated the AIDS group program." Shaking his head in disbelief, "Disability. The only job I'll have now is cashing disability checks. I no longer have a social work job." The cadence of Jason's voice and his anger quickened. "I can't believe it! They knew all the group leaders had AIDS. They hired us, that was the criteria. Now they let us go because our symptoms are more obvious. They went ahead and ended the program."

Neil became indignant, "That's outrageous! We need more caretakers, not fewer. I can't believe the hospital let you go. They don't get it, do they? If caregivers get eliminated, we get eliminated."

Matthew joined in, "The system doesn't leave any option except activism. We need more caretakers, and to Jason's point, there's going to be more of us. That's the whole issue Vito's been talking about. Activists go to ACT UP, therapists to GMHC, and social workers run AIDS groups in hospitals."

Jason's voice deepened, "I heard a nurse at the hospital say it was a real pain to keep replacing us group leaders. 'Take care of yourself,' one of the doctors told me after I got laid off." Jason mumbled, "Running groups *was* taking care of myself!" He shot a painful glance in my direction.

Finally, I heard what Jason hadn't said. "Jason, we both know, and the group knows that you've been co-leading *this* group since the beginning. That doesn't make up for what the hospital did and co-leading with me is certainly different from having your own group, but you and I have been working together since the group began." I paused, "I've got to tell you, when GMHC agreed I could solo lead a group, that was crazy. You know so much more about AIDS than I do, about symptoms, medications. It was in our very first session when you took the reins, and said, 'no one here dies.'"

Jason stared at the floor, shifted around on his folding chair, and sighed, "I think this is a good time to end the session. Do you agree?"

Was he in agreement that he was co-leading with me, or did my comment make him feel defeated? I couldn't tell. If I asked him, he might feel shamed if his answer was 'defeated.' I mean, I took the wind out of his sails. Does that feel like relief from anger, or does that feel dead in the water? How do you comfort a dying man who has just been fired, and then told by a doctor he's no longer needed?

"Yes," I whispered. "It's a perfect time to end."

Chapter 15
In the Beginning...

Jason's question, 'Why am I leading an AIDS group therapy' and 'why am I still here,' was insightful. At the time, I only credited superficial reasons, such as providing referrals and building a private practice. To be honest as well as embarrassed, I was well into writing this book before the real reasons came into awareness. It wasn't that I forgot the memories in this chapter, rather my unconscious was just overly perfecting two ego defenses, denial and blocking.

It was in early 1970s, before moving to New York City, that I apprenticed in Summer Stock theater in Ohio. While there, I became close friends with two other apprentices, both were gay men, Billy and Greg. The three of us agreed to move to NYC that September. Our thinking was that we would provide support for each other, thus allowing emotional freedom enroute to Broadway theatre stardom.

Upon arrival in NYC, Billy and Greg got a great Upper Westside apartment. I rented a room from a British woman who had two enormous cats and a gorgeous gay guy roommate. The apartment was an old tenement building in Greenwich Village, Third Street and MacDougal.

The British woman, the gorgeous gay guy, and I shared a four hundred square foot apartment on the top floor. The toilet was down the hall, unusual but not unheard of back then and we three shared it with two other apartments on the same floor. The shower was not near the bathroom, but rather in the kitchen and believe me, way too narrow for a soap dish. One evening, the British woman made dinner for us. Meatloaf with a banana in the center. She explained the banana kept the meatloaf moist. I remember the meatloaf. I don't remember the moist.

It was almost instantaneous that Greg got a job in the Costume Department of a prestigious Broadway Theatre. Billy was hired as a Stage Manager and over time worked for both Broadway and Off-Broadway productions. Greg and Billy were rarely out of work, which is an oddity in the theatre world.

Unfortunately, the only acting job I secured was nowhere near Broadway. I was hired as a typist and had to *act* as though I knew how. In the 1970s, there were many entry-level jobs for women without a college education. I had a high school degree, nothing more. The only job I was marginally qualified for was receptionist, but those jobs were hard to get. The easiest job was secretary. Naturally, we were required to take typing tests before getting hired. My typing test score was twenty-five typed-words-a-minute with twenty or so mistakes. Surprisingly, this was good enough for an advertising agency. They hired me as a secretary/typist. Who would have guessed advertising agencies needed secretaries who couldn't type. In addition to typing, I landed a lead role in an Off-Off Broadway show. Unfortunately, the experience didn't hold the excitement I anticipated, and I spent more money traveling to rehearsals than I made at the advertising agency.

While Billy was doing well getting stage-managing jobs, Greg went from sewing costumes to Costume Director in a New-York-Minute. He befriended famous Broadway stars during costume fittings and was soon socially elevated to the top people in theatre.

Greg was perfect for the theatre world. He was a sensationally spectacular stunning gay man with the Irish gift of storytelling. He had long curly light blonde hair, a six-pack stomach and beautiful body that excelled in turning gay men's heads. Actually, his beauty whiplashed their heads.

In addition to collecting Broadway stars, Greg quickly gathered a gorgeous galaxy of gay men into his universe. Let's face it, Billy and I were delighted because neither of us had any problem being in a mob of men. One of Greg's first admirers was a mildly-almost sort-of attractive guy, Alex. Unfortunately, Alex couldn't make headway into Greg's adoring circle/bed. However, rather than give up, Alex changed tact, claimed bisexuality, and pursued me. I soon realized the bisexual claim was a ruse. This realization came after Alex told me that's why we were dating. Still, Alex took me dancing at Studio 54 and no surprise, he invited Greg who was 'busy but might show up.' This 'might show' excuse kept Alex dating me longer than he initially intended.

It was a little embarrassing that Billy and Greg got theatre jobs and I didn't, but one must audition before one is cast in a show. At least I had my typing job. While licking my wounds, I signed up for acting classes where I learned how to enunciate with a wine cork lodged between upper and lower teeth. I also learned how to fall without incurring injuries. This skill comes in handy if you get hired for a stunt job in the movies. In addition, I have found the falling down skill has become quite helpful as I get older. Anyway, my scene partner in acting class was a breathtaking beautiful gay man who over time introduced me to his friends, all of whom were gay. Yes, the scene we performed for our acting class was *Streetcar Named Desire.*

As a result, for the first three to five years in New York, I usually hung out with gay men. They were way easier to befriend than straight women in my typing pool. I assume these typing pool women thought they were better than me, especially when it came to typing. So, for a few years, I was either with Greg and/or Billy and their gay friends, or I was with my acting school scene-partner and his gay friends.

After finishing/quitting Acting School, I came up with a rationale for terminating my theatrical career: 1) I was too nervous to audition and therefore never did; 2) I feared starving to death without a day job; 3) if I stayed in theatre, I'd probably end up marrying a gay guy because straight men in theatre are scarce. On the other hand, this was a fallacy because Greg's gay/bisexual friend, Alex, eventually dumped me, meaning I had a bleak future of even marrying a gay or bisexual theatre guy. Billy and Greg, however, remained in theatre and I kept my finger on the Broadway pulse by purchasing single-seat tickets, "Just one, please." Or buying (SRO) Standing Room Only, which meant floor space for your own two feet, for $3.00.

Greg, as I mentioned was no dim bulb on Broadway. He was making good money in various Broadway Theater

Costume Departments. I, too, liked to sew, however, my sewing skill ran neck and neck with my typing ability. At any rate, Billy and I benefited from Greg's massively increasing famous-people connections, similar to our benefiting from Greg's galaxy of gay men. As luck would have it, Greg's costume career provided Billy and me with free tickets for whatever Broadway show Greg was sewing. We saw *Pacific Overtures*, *A Chorus Line*, *A Little Night Music*, *Chicago,* and a bunch of 'straight' plays, no oxymoron. Greg's stardom also provided Billy and I with backstage entry where we 'saw' Michael Bennett. This sighting lasted for one split second after curtain call for *A Chorus Line*. I'm pretty sure it was Bennett, but I don't actually know what Bennett looks like.

As I mentioned previously, Greg's theatre contacts helped him slide right into the fast-paced, sexually active, chic drug-using, New York City theatre aristocrat circles. He also joined New York City Gay Men's Chorus. In hindsight, I wonder if he attended the New York City Gay Men's Chorus 'Night at the Movies' that Vito hosted.

Concurrent with Greg's star-is-born metro-phoric rise, he became less and less available to me and Billy. However, I was achieving my own stardom having progressed to way fewer typing errors. After a while, I sought my second acting role. Who knew publishing houses as well as advertising agencies hire typists who can't type.

During my stint at the publishing job, my yearly income shot up to $8,000.00, just a smidgen over the poverty line. However, this publishing house had a lot of perks, such as an eighty percent medical reimbursement policy. As a result, I went to therapy twice a week with a lovely therapist. She set me straight about my future as a typist. I was now twenty-eight years old with only a high school education and no idea what I wanted to do with my life. One day my therapist asked, 'If you could do anything, what might it be?' I responded, "I want to do what you do."

"Okay," she said. "Do this: Go to college and stay there until you have a doctorate. Then, go to a four-year psychoanalytic training institute and get a certificate in psychoanalysis and psychotherapy."

"I'll do just that." Quite a few (many) years later, I had my PhD and a Certificate in Psychoanalysis.

Throughout this time, Billy and I stayed in touch even though we had gone different directions. He continued stage-managing and supplemented his income with an Off-Broadway job as a landscaper for New York City rooftop terraces. He told me landscaping penthouse terraces was akin to designing stage backdrops. I agreed with him even though I didn't. Slowly, over the next eight years we saw less and less of Greg. As time went on, Billy got used to having an absentee roommate who paid rent and was never there. There are few New Yorkers who would take exception to this roommate arrangement.

Then, one evening in 1980, Billy phoned, "I need you to sit down."

"Why?"

"Listen." Billy's deep voice pitched and cracked, "Greg passed away?"

"What? What? What do you mean?"

"Greg's dead."

"What do you mean he's dead?"

"He contracted parasites."

"What in the hell are parasites?" This parasites diagnosis was the maiden name for AIDS. In the early 1980s, many of us began receiving emotional calls from gay friends about other gay friends who were dying from 'euphemistic illnesses.' A few years later, AIDS had its rightful name and chosen population.

"Tom passed away."

"What? I just saw him on his sitcom last week."

"They filmed that a while ago."

"Oh, no. Don't tell me. AIDS?"

"Yes."

A few months later another gay friend called, "Hey, I wanted to tell you that Juan died."

"Juan died? AIDS?"

Another group of months passed, "Marvin's being buried next week."

"What? We had lunch about six months ago. Oh, maybe it was more than six months ago. AIDS, right?"

Weeks later, the phone rang. "Do you want to join us for a memorial service for David."

"Oh, no. No. Nooooo."

"I know," he whispered back. "We're meeting at the Monster Bar, Sheridan Square at 7:00. You should come, it might be the last time you'll see Doug and Aaron. They're both pretty sick."

"I'll be there. Oh, Billy's been with his family in Wisconsin for a while, but if he's back I'll invite him."

"You don't have to call Billy."

"Why? Billy's fine. He doesn't have AIDS. His AIDS test was negative. He just went home to help his dad run the family business. You're wrong. Billy doesn't have AIDS.

He told me he doesn't have AIDS. Are we talking about the same Billy?"

If you took the test too early after exposure, the results could reveal a false negative.

This was how the plague began. This is how it continued…

Chapter 16
The Little Black Book

On this Wednesday evening, everyone was here, including our famous guy, Vito, who was briefly home from lecturing and teaching. In the beginning of this session, Vito was a little subdued, distracted. It took about ten minutes before he spoke up. "Listen, there's something I need to talk about. Something important to me, very important." The pink baseball-ish cap inhaled and Vito began. "Alright," his voice cracked. "I just lost another friend yesterday and I'm pissed. I'm so damn angry." Vito's body shivered as his eyes opened wider than I thought possible. He looked around scanning everyone's face.

"Nobody dies. You all made that pledge. Jason, right? Look, I can't lose more people. I can't keep stockpiling emptiness, sadness, death. The more people I lose, the hollower I feel, and the more my anger skyrockets." He folded his hands on his lap. "Why?" he asked, frustration increasing. "Why are we still dying?" He looked around, "When I die, there might not be any friends at my funeral. They'll all be dead."

I watched Vito's finger gently tap his shirt pocket, then pull out a little black address book. He shook his head as he flipped each page. For a moment, he stopped to stare at it, then quickly turned the address book in our direction. His hands shook from anger. "See this?" He started turning each page, one by one. The entries, the names and addresses of Vito's friends were scribbled over, blacked out. "Almost every single entry, every line." Vito looked at us while furiously shaking the book. "This, this is my life. These people." He cleared his throat, "These people, my friends, they should be alive. My people. I loved them." He slammed the book on his knee, then, as though the address book had a name, he uttered, "Jeffery."

Richard looked panic-stricken, "Why do you carry that around?" No answer. Vito's expression seemed a silent demand, a renewal of, 'no one here dies.' His fingers slid over the leather address book. Perhaps soothing his lost friends. Then, returned it to his shirt pocket.

"To answer your question, Richard, about why I carry this book around." Vito's eyes moistened, "If I throw this book away, I'm throwing them away. As long as I have this, I have them."

I panicked, "Am I the only one here with alive people in my address book? Do the rest of them have address books like Vito's? When they scratch out a name, do they worry about their name being scribbled over?"

The entirety of this session focused on everyone's black address books, all with inked-over names. I was right. My address book was the sole survivor, albeit minus many of my gay friends.

At some point, I looked down at my watch and realized my preoccupation prematurely pushed me to the edge of my folding chair. My anxiety was sky high. I forgot what time it was from the previous second after I checked my watch. I pushed myself back on the chair. *"Ten more minutes,"* I thought. No, I can't do ten more minutes. Thank goodness, Jason was still able to hear the unspoken, "I think we should stop for today."

"Yes, I think we should stop. We only have ten more minutes left anyway, it's time," I announced, as though it was my job to end the session, which at this point, I didn't care whose job it was.

A few men stood up to leave. A few shrugged or shifted as though they weren't sure what to do. Some of the guys seemed emotionally nonexistent and a couple of them looked stuck to their chair. No words, no disagreements or agreements to leave or not. After a few long minutes, they were gone.

Chapter 17
Guilt

Once, when I was visiting Budapest, I decided to walk the ramparts of the Buda castle to view the historic city. My stroll began with the end of a light rainfall leaving the rampart walls glistening. As I walked, I could see deep scars embedded by invaders, conquerors, or protectors warding off foreign oppression. My fingers followed the wall, like a stick dragged across a picket fence only interrupted by an occasional crescent peaked copula. Approaching one, I heard singing. A young woman standing inside a copula, singing a gypsy folk song of exile. The purity of her voice and the sad poetry of the music seemed to deepen the rampart scars. She sang about forgotten lives, about prejudice of differences, about loss of what will never be. Meager remains of a culture never absorbed.

Sometimes during our Wednesday night sessions, the men spoke about a future that would not include them. They talked about the government and the public being prejudice because this was a 'gay disease.' They spoke about the FDA holding back approval of necessary medications leaving gay men to feel they are disposable. They worried about their family's reactions to their death. Who will be mourned, who won't be missed. Their discussions sometimes focused on their family's financial struggles from the cost of AZT and how to sell their life insurance to reimburse relatives. Eight gay men often spoke of feeling helpless to alter an all-too-soon finality as well as weighted guilt of surviving when others died.

A few men in my group, like Thomas, had discussed their family's reaction when told they had AIDS. Some group members were further rejected, some were brought closer to the fold. Others lamented never having opportunity to know the next generation; children not yet born to their families. A few worried if their lovers would replace them with new lovers.

There were also narratives about missing themselves, who they used to be before physical deterioration. Suicide was not an uncommon topic. Why waste away when they could control the end, save family money, and eliminate their excruciating pain. Suicide meant no more expenditures for AZT, no more money spent on hospital bills or mental health costs. A few of my men talked about the best way to achieve a successful suicide.

This is a professional and ethical conundrum. Therapists are meant to inhibit suicide. Thankfully, no one in my group prematurely took his own life. Still, I have wondered what was moral in this particular time of AIDS?

Chapter 18
The Socratic Method

"I'd like to talk about hemlock," Jason announced at the beginning of the next session.

Richard's voice pitched as he slid forward on his folding chair. "You're thinking about using that? Hemlock? Are you going to the Hemlock Society?"

Jason paused, then looked at Richard who continued, "Are you seriously thinking about hemlock?"

"No, but a friend of mine is."

"Did he use it?"

"No." Jason had a way with sarcasm, "It'd be hard for him to tell me about it, if he'd already used it."

Richard's curiosity and voice spiked, "Isn't it painful to drink? Socrates was in a lot of pain after he used it."

"Richard." Jason teased, "I get the feeling, you don't want any."

"Right. I don't want any." Richard's body retreated, as though Jason was about to hand him a goblet. "What if you take it too soon? What if somebody drinks it and changes his mind? What if someone drank it and the next day they developed a cure serum for AIDS?"

"Richard, you should put off hemlock as long as possible," Chris chimed in.

"Oh, definitely," Richard retorted. "Yeah, I'd put off hemlock, for sure. But, Jason, if you need help or money to purchase hemlock, let me know."

Tongue in cheek, "Not a problem. I've lined up an expert in hemlock drinking so it goes down smoothly with a spoonful of sugar."

Jason took a quick breath before Richard could interrupt again. "Look. My friend, the guy who is considering hemlock, is in bad shape. He's in unbelievable pain, nerve pain."

Fernando sighed, "Our lives are already short and your friend wants to make his even shorter. His pain must be excruciating."

"Yeah. Who knows if he'll get some or if he'll use it."

"You need a lot of courage to drink that," Thomas mumbled. "Never mind. I'll take that back. Pain creates courage."

"I plan to be around as long as I can," Matthew lamented.

Richard wasn't satisfied. "So, what is it that happens if you drink hemlock?"

Jason inhaled, "You feel poisoned and then you die. Your nervous system goes first, Richard. My friend sold his life insurance and paid all his medical bills. His partner died a couple years ago and my friend is ready to join him. He wants to go home to Hawaii."

"Why Hawaii?" Fernando gingerly questioned.

"His family lives there for one thing. Also, I think burial laws in Hawaii are lenient. A while ago, he mentioned native born Hawaiians could be buried in unmarked places on the Islands. Doesn't matter if the remains are bones or ashes."

Without missing a beat, Jason anticipated Richard's next question, "I don't know anything more about Hawaiian burials, Richard. That's all I know."

Richard nodded, cleared his throat, slid to the edge of his chair, leaned forward, and excitedly bopped around a little, then inquired, "So, getting back to the point, how much does hemlock cost?"

Fernando reacted, "Richard, you're nowhere near buying hemlock."

Attempting an end or interrupting the hemlock conversation, Neil jumped in, "Oh, I forgot! I have to miss next week. My mother asked me to come home, just for a week. I'll miss next session."

Jason leaned into my hair/left ear, and under his breath, "Jesus, his mother lost her husband when Neil was little. Now she'll lose Neil."

I sighed, "Can't imagine what that feels like to lose both husband and son."

Jason softly whispered, "You'll see."

Chapter 19
Thomas' Pain

Entering the session room the following week, I quickly grabbed my seat after I heard Thomas announce, "There's something I want to discuss tonight. Well, first I'd better say I went home over the weekend. I wanted to visit my mother and my sister. I know that meant seeing my father, but I miss my mother and my sister. When I was home, I thought about that session when Neil talked about his father. The part about his father being on the *Kittyhawk* and how he died trying to land the plane." We all nodded 'yes' as encouragement. Thomas shook his head, "Neil thinks about his father so differently than I do about mine."

Thomas stared at the ceiling, then sarcastically added, "Disappointment." Thomas' mood was visibly darkening, "The first disappointment was my birth. I never told you guys that I was a twin. Two boys, and according to dear old dad, I was so big there was no room for my twin. Maybe my twin was going to be the perfect son. Growing up, my mother and I became close. She was probably afraid she might lose me, too."

"When I was around five, I knew I was different. I think my mother knew early on, too. At some point, she told my dad I might be gay. He was so upset that she back peddled and said she must be wrong." Exasperated, "When I'm about six or seven, kids start calling me a sissy. My dad heard about this, probably from the guidance counselor and he jumps on the band wagon calling me a sissy. He wanted to make me into a man. A man at seven years old. So, he insisted I play football. I'm seven! I am not going to play football. 'Then play basketball.' No, I'm still seven. I'm not going to play basketball."

"Once he said to me, 'Who made you gay?' Unbelievable, he said that. Then he says, 'Your mother made you gay. Don't tell me she didn't.' Fast forward to now, because here I am, trying to spend time with my mother and sister. Just us girls. It's like he's jealous. We're not giving him enough attention, and I've finally had it. I told them to leave the room, that I wanted to talk to Dad. So now I'm alone with my father. He's spitting angry that I made his audience leave. Like I said, I'm tired of holding it together and I belt out, 'You're miserable and you want us to be just as miserable.'"

Thomas shook his head, "Once again, we're at it, just like old times. At some point, he yells for my mother. He calls her 'Mother.' Not 'Jill.' 'Mother.' He wants his audience back and he wants my mother and sister to be there and be miserable. I know he wants me to leave because that'll concretize everyone's misery. 'Mother,' he yells. 'Come here. Now!' Of course she comes back. Whatever he wants her to do, she does. Of course, he keeps shouting even though by now she's in the same room. 'It's your fault,' he says to her. 'I warned you about coddling him. You hovered over him. You didn't want him to go to away to school because you'd miss him too much.' Then, he looks at me and shouts, 'That's why I sent you away as soon as I could, so she wouldn't make you into more of a sissy.' Then he says to my mother, 'This family has fallen apart and it your fault.' She starts apologizing, 'I'm so sorry. I'm sorry.' Thomas mimicked his father's voice, 'You'd better be sorry.' Then Dad turns to me, 'Don't touch anything. You'll give us AIDS. You're not wanted here. You and your virus.'"

Fernando interrupted, "Your father is a monster. He's cruel. How in the world did you grow up normal?"

"I grew up in boarding schools, thank you Dad. He scared my mother to the degree she was afraid to hug me when I left that day. Not because I've got AIDS. It's because he'd blast her if she disobeyed him." Thomas' body slumped, weary after his diatribe.

"Oh god, I know what that's like. 'Don't touch him! You'll get AIDS!'" Matthew said mockingly.

Vito interrupted, "So do I. I know exactly what you're talking about. When I'm going on TV, the make-up people are afraid to touch me."

"Unbelievable," Fernando reacted loudly.

Matthew threw up his hands, "It's incredible. A lot of people think if they're in the same room, they'll get 'infected." He smirked, "Let me tell you, it'd be a catastrophe if I pricked my finger pinning clothes on mannequins for the store's windows. The girls would flip out and get an AIDS test."

Jason laughed sardonically, "I remember when straight men thought gays would force them to have sex."

Vito retorted, "It's amazing. We are going to seduce straight men because there aren't enough gays to go around. Jesus, we're always predators, outsiders, undesirables. Now, it's worse, right? We'll force them to have sex and give them AIDS. Seriously, can you imagine me or any one of us, being strong enough to force a straight guy to have sex?"

"I know!" Thomas echoed. "Damn, I remember this one time, I was home from university and my dad's friends, their children were getting engaged, getting married, and I wasn't doing either."

Fernando interrupted, "They were probably pregnant before they married, right?" Sarcastically Fernando continued, "Well, when I told my parents I was gay, my father looks at me like I've got two heads, 'Why did you *go* gay?' '*Go* gay?' Like I made a wrong decision. 'Go gay?' Right, I'm gay out of spite?"

In a resigned tone, Matthew commented, "My father wasn't happy either but not that bad. He said I should go to therapy. It might make me straight. As though I should make a U-turn and go straight."

Matthew looked at me, "You don't turn people straight, do you? Do you believe someone gay can become straight?"

"Hell, no!" I said dramatically, surprised at my own emotionality.

Matthew continued, "Didn't Freud think he could do that?"

"No. Where you getting that from? Okay, wait a minute." I put up my hand like a traffic cop. "Listen, I know many people have misconceptions about Freud, but they probably haven't read his work. They've most likely read a secondary source; an article written *about* Freud, not Freud's publications. Secondary sources can be biased, one way or another, and then you're reading someone else's opinion and not Freud's own work. I'm not Freudian; that's Traditional or Classical psychoanalysis. I'm a Contemporary psychoanalyst. Relational analysis." I scanned their faces. They all looked like I was speaking Celtiberian,

"Never mind, it's too much to explain. Bottom line, if it wasn't for Freud, we wouldn't have psychology. As far as Freud's thoughts about homosexuality, do you know about the letter he wrote to an American woman? She wanted Freud to make her son straight. Freud wrote back and told her many individuals can be sexually attracted to both women and men. It's a natural outcome of relationships. He said some of the greatest people in history have been gay, Alexander the Great, Plato, Michelangelo, Leonardo da Vinci, Proust, Oscar Wilde, Rock Hudson, Elton John." You could have heard a pin drop, except my smirk gave me away.

Immediately, laughter filled the room, "Freud knew Elton John? Rock Hudson?" Chris' red curls were dancing like crazy.

I joked, "Oh, absolutely! Freud knew Elton. He played base in Elton's band. I wasn't there, so actually I'm not positive it was base guitar." It was nice to make my men smile.

Richard interrupted, "Can we get back to the topic?"

"I don't think she strayed, Richard. She's talking about rejection; about being gay and rejected," Chris chimed in.

"I'm glad my dad didn't react like yours, Thomas," Matthew interjected. "I got to say, I love him, and I love my mother. My dad made sure we had a good life. We grew up in a great neighborhood and we had nice house."

Matthew's tone turned melodic, "It was a very beautiful old house. Victorian." He shot a glance at me. "You're mentioning Freud, the Victorian area, made me think of it. My house is painted white with dark green shutters, the original shutters. It was built in the 1850s. Tons of windows, one is a funny oval shape with stained glass."

Out of the blue, Thomas shot right through Matthew's mood. He must have been ruminating about his father and picked up where he'd left off, "Before he threw me out of the house, my dad yelled, 'You should have loved me, not them. You loved your mother. Your sister. Never me. If you'd have loved me, you'd be straight."

We were all taken aback by Thomas' statement.

Thomas shook his head in disbelief, "Did any of you ever read *Washington Square*?"

"Yes," I almost said, then realized it was a rhetorical question.

"Henry James wrote it. It's about a woman who falls in love with the wrong man. According to my father, I fell in love with the wrong man." He scoffed, "How ironic, the 'wrong man.' My father is the wrong man," Thomas was livid, sadly livid.

Richard interrupted, "I don't get it. It sounds like he threw temper tantrums, you know, like yelling and intimidating your mother. I mean, your father is weird."

"Spot on, Richard," Thomas confirmed, then looked at me or maybe it was Jason, "It's time to go home, don't you think?"

"Yup, we're done. See you all next week," Jason replied. He was looking at Jason.

Chapter 20
Down Mexico Way

A few weeks later, the moment Fernando arrived, he announced, "Porque hace frio afuera! Necesito el clima cálido de México!"

"I don't know what you said, but if you're going to Mexico, I'm going with you," Jason joked.

Chris jumped in, "Where? Yucatan?"

"No, no, too many New Yorkers." Fernando smiled and continued, "I'm go to Cuernavaca. Beautiful Cuernavaca. You guys ever been there?"

"Oh, I've been there," Neil declared.

"Hey, Neil. You're back." Fernando seemed surprised he hadn't noticed Neil's presence. "Missed you last week."

"Missed you guys, too." Neil responded, then added, "It's such a fantastic city, a bedroom community close to Mexico City, Central Mexico. Absolutely beautiful. When I was there, the hotel we stayed at was fabulous. Flowers all over the place, exotic plants everywhere, deep green lush lawns. I remember the grass was so thick they swept it with a broom." He looked around, some of the guys looked incredulous. "No, really, I felt it! It was real grass."

Fernando laughed, "He's right, they sweep the grass. When the flower pedals or leaves fall to the ground, the brooms come out."

"They don't vacuum?" Jason quipped.

"That'd be an enormous vacuum, Jason. Yes, Neil, it is a beautiful city," Fernando happily replied. "It's magnificent. Full of Bougainvillea. Every color Bougainvillea you can think of, everywhere. So many historic buildings and the Aztec ruins are there. Some excavated and some just a little. Mexico City is built on the ruins of Tenochtitlan, the capital of the Aztec Empire."

"I knew that!" Richard exclaimed.

Attempting to encourage Fernando, I pursued, "Well, tell us more." I nodded to Richard for confirmation that I hadn't cut him off. Until this moment, I didn't realize Richard had gotten so thin. I glanced at Jason; did he see this too? Amidst glancing, I was taken aback. Jason looked exhausted and I realized he was just as thin as Richard. I turned to him, worried, "You okay?" I didn't say that out loud. Jason gave me a small smile. He was still astute at hearing the unspoken.

"Fernando, did you grow up there?" Thomas asked.

"No, here. But my father and mother did, they grew up in Cuernavaca. My father's family are flower farmers. Their flowers are sold everywhere. All over the world."

Richard interrupted, "How often do you see your family if they live in Mexico?"

"My parents and my older brother moved to California before I was born. They bought a flower farm."

"They bought a flower farm in California with money from growing flowers in Mexico? What'd they grow? Poppies?" Chris teased.

Chris could say anything to anyone in the group and no one took offense. Now that I think about it, that's entirely true.

Fernando continued, "No, no poppies. My father wanted his own flower farm. He brought some relatives up from Mexico to help. When we were old enough, we helped. We worked before school and after." Fernando shook his head, "Oh, yeah, and you'd better get good grades."

Thomas was inquisitive, "Did they speak English when they moved here?"

"My father did, yeah. My dad worked hard and we all lived well."

"It's just you and your brother?" Chris asked.

"Nope. I have four sisters, two older and two younger, my brother is the oldest. I'm the fourth kid, in the middle of the girls."

Neil commented, "Were you closer to your older or younger sisters?"

Fernando mused, "My older sisters took care of me. They took care of all the kids before we were old enough to help on the farm."

"Your sisters were younger than your older brother, right? Why didn't he take care of all of you?" Richard asked.

"Nah, not my brother, Emilio. He was destined for greater things. He was really good at sports, even as a kid. He made All Star his senior year in high school. Not me. No sports. Just like you, Thomas. Why should I play sports. No way would I even begin to compete with my brother. He's a natural athletic."

Fernando stopped, took a deep breath, then continued, "When I finished high school, I left the farm and came to New York. My father didn't want me to leave." Imitating his father's voice, 'You work *here*,' he said. Fernando's voice pitched, "My brother went to college. My father wanted Emilio to play professional sports." Fernando scoffed, "I went to college, but I had to come home on weekends to help. After I graduated, I told my dad I wanted to go to New York. He said, 'If you leave here, you'll get nothing from me.'" Exasperated, Fernando added, "So, I hitchhiked from California to New York and got no help from my dad."

Thomas interrupted, "You showed him."

"I wish I'd showed him with some of his money in my pocket. When I got here, I stayed with a friend in the projects. The projects on the upper eastside." Fernando looked around, "You want to get material for a book? Live in the projects for a while."

"What happened?" Richard was on the edge of his chair.

"You know what those places are like, right? They're full of people struggling with life. Some have almost nothing. Lots of kids and very little furniture. Drugs are everywhere. Oh, and you definitely want to take the stairs if you can, because the elevators smell. I remember hearing a bunch of guys talking about doing crack and shooting heroin. They were sort of bragging about how many times they overdosed on heroin. As though being brought back to life held some sort of status. Some of them get money for drugs by turning in empty soda cans from the garbage. They know when and where garbage trucks pick up stuff and they'd get there early before the garbage guys took it. Hell, it must have been a hay day for them during the garbage strikes a couple of years ago."

Jason chimed in, "Oh yeah, that was awful. We had the garbage strike almost right after the transit strike."

Matthew laughed, "Oh, my god, you should have seen the weird fashions during the transit strike."

"I'd like to get back to Fernando's experience," Richard broke in.

Fernando chuckled, "Sure. Well, it didn't take long to get a job in the flower district downtown because I know about flowers. That made it easy to talk with the wholesale buyers. I got a couple of offers to work in florist shops, but you know, they didn't want to pay more than what I was already making. I turned them down until this one guy came in. He had a flower shop on the Eastside in the 60s. He wasn't a regular. He came because his buyer was out sick. Well, this guy was wearing an ascot and a double-breasted blazer, ventless."

"Whoa! Ventless!" Matthew joked.

Fernando grinned, "Well, Mr. Ascot saw I knew a lot about flowers and made me an offer. He told me how much money I'd make if I worked for him. Then somehow, we got to talking about where I lived, and I told him I was temporarily staying with a friend in the projects." Fernando smiled, "I think he wanted to save me from the projects because he said I could stay in the apartment above his shop. That's where he lived. I would have my own private room and if I worked in the shop, I'd pay very little rent. So I jumped at it and moved in. True to his word, I got my own room." Fernando inhaled, "After a while, we realized we liked each other and about a month or so later, we were in love. It turns out the flower shop was sort of his plaything. His family had money, which meant the apartment above the florist shop was huge! His name was Max, Maximilian. I called him Maxie. He loved that. He was in his forties. A great body, handsome enough. He sort of greened me."

Richard asked, "What do you mean?"

"Well, he took me on trips to Europe. We went to museums, and he knew a lot about art." Fernando sheepishly looked down. "I'd never seen a real Rembrandt before Maxie, but now I know about Rembrandt's brush strokes." Fernando mused, "Maxie loved good food and we went to phenomenal restaurants in Paris, Rome, Venice, all over Europe and of course, New York. He had season tickets for the Philharmonic, and for the ballet. I don't know how Maxie did it, but this one time, for my birthday he arranged for us to watch a ballet class. David Howard was teaching. You won't believe this. Baryshnikov was taking this class. Nice guy. A little short, but nice guy."

"Anyway, Maxie taught me everything. How to *be* in the world and appreciate what life has to offer; the art of living, in a way." Fernando sat straighter, "Whenever we travelled it was first class. I loved Italy. I could live there." Fernando leaned back on his folding chair, "Maxie died three years ago from the virus. I inherited his shop, but I sold it. It felt like I was surrounded by Maxie, like I was living in his belly."

I commiserated, "It's like he's everywhere. Too many overwhelming reminders of who he was. Who you were together, and now, what you've lost and won't forget."

Fernando looked surprised. "How do you know? Did this happen to you?"

"Of course," I whispered. "How else would I know? I probably felt just a small piece of what you experienced, though. I know about losing love." What I really meant and did not say, "I will lose eight men who inhabit my inner world. I know what I will lose, and I know I'll never forget."

They were quiet. Probably in reaction to my vulnerability. For the first time, I felt their tenderness, their warmth. For the first time, my vulnerability made me more acceptable.

No one spoke for a minute or so, until Richard interrupted, "Where do you live now? I mean besides living in Maxie's belly."

Fernando smiled at me, then turned to Richard, "Soho."

"Didn't you inherit money, too?"

"No, just the shop. Maxie's money was in a Trust. It went back into his family's Trust." Fernando signed, "I didn't want to own the shop. Too much stress. I mean I ran the shop after Maxie got sick. I did that until he passed. That was enough." Fernando face flushed, "I miss him. You know? I really miss him."

Thomas gently interrupted, "You've had a life of contradictory experiences. A flower farm in California, living in the projects in Manhattan, and then seeing the world differently through Maxie."

"Yeah, I *had* a good life."

We were all encompassed by the emotionality within Fernando, until Richard once again disrupted the mood.

"Talking about family. I have a family reunion next week. I'll try to come back alive."

Chapter 21
Cheerleading

It is now 1989. Absent: Richard is at a family reunion. Vito is teaching at a university in California.

Chris was one of the younger members of the group, probably in his early twenties and without question, the most visibly vibrant. He was easy to like; personable, humorous, emotionally present, and very empathic. In addition, it seemed we all admired his curly red hair and appreciated its involvement during our discussions. For example, let's say Chris is telling a story and at the right moment a curl or two could jump right down onto his forehead like a comma, semi-colon, or sometimes a question mark. It was adorable, watching his red curls play on his beautiful porcelain skin; that see-through sheer bone-china color skin. Just like the wedding present china you put on display in the never-used-dining-room cabinet because 'what if somebody broke it.' That was Chris.

He wasn't just fascinating to look at, there was a showmanship about Chris, as you know. He was artistically talented, skilled, a natural born entertainer. Chris was a wonderful dancer/singer on Broadway and was so talented he was usually went from one musical play to the next.

Chris sometimes spoke about the choreographers he knew, his tap and jazz dance classes, and his singing lessons.

"Theater must pay pretty well to have money for all those classes," Fernando noted.

"Not really. My mother helped." Chris shrugged, "Most mothers would do the same."

"You've got a special mother, Chris," Thomas expressed.

"My mother is like that, too." Matthew chimed in.

Chris' curls became quite animated after Fernando's compliment. It was mesmerizing. Chris continued, "My mother is something else. She used to be a model with Ford Modeling Agency right up until she married my father. Thank goodness I inherited my hair from the maternal line."

"What was it like growing up with a model mother. I mean a mother who modeled. The only models I know are not mothers." The window dresser in Matthew leaned forward, perhaps hoping to hear classified department-store information from a model's perspective.

Chris smiled, "She paid a price for being pretty because my dad thought every man was after her and that was part of why they got divorced. She had to travel a lot, sometimes to Europe. My father was extremely jealous and accused her of having affairs whenever she travelled. Of course, it was my dad who was having affairs and when she found out, she filed for divorced. I guess I was around five when he left." Chris lowered his head as red curls cascaded forward, just like the theatre's red velvet curtain dismissing Act 1.

"Keep going, Chris," Matthew insisted.

"Yeah, what happened next?" Thomas asked.

"Well," Chris sat up straighter and pushed back his curls, the red curtain rising again. "My mom took a full-time job when he left. She was offered a good position at the modeling agency."

Did she have to know how to type? No one heard me think that, including Jason. Everyone was engaged and relaxed as Chris continued his story. I mean, let's face it, Chris could make any narrative come alive, even an Easter hat.

"Eventually my mom became head of Personnel, which meant I was a latch key kid in elementary school. When I got to high school, I joined every after-school activity, so I wouldn't be alone waiting for my mother." Chris joked, "Not sports, though. Not the Chess Club, and definitely not the Rod and Gun Club." He chuckled, "You'll love this part. There was one activity that took up a lot of after-school time, cheerleading. I became the third male cheerleader at our school. My mother was thrilled!" Chris and his red curls looked like Chinese New Year firecrackers on Mott Street.

My mind went like arms akimbo. I imagined Chris and his red curls, jumping around the basketball court or the football field, cheerleading like crazy. I didn't make Cheerleading. You have to audition in order to get in, and you know by now I was audition-challenged. However, I did make the Girl's Drill Team. No auditions. They weren't picky. Our Drill Team had rifles made of wood, painted powder blue and white, our school colors. We wore majorette boots with tap-dancing cleats on them and we performed 'drills' in local parades. There we were, swinging our powder blue and white wood rifles in circles and taping majorette boots on asphalt.

"Your school had boy cheerleaders?" Neil seemed a tad envious.

"We did, Neil, and thank goodness. It was the only almost-sport I was good at. A little like dancing." Chris' curls grinned in delight. "A friend told me we should take ballet classes because it'd help our cheerleading ability. So we signed up for ballet and jazz classes and I was hooked. It was all about cheerleading and dance from then on."

Thomas' curiosity peaked, "Your mother was okay with your being a dancer and a cheerleader. She must have known you were gay, right?"

Chris' curls shook 'no.' "She probably knew, but there was no discussion. Besides, she thought dancing and cheerleading were safer than football." Chris was becoming more animated. "Those football guys scared the hell out of me. Oh god, I remember once I was cheerleading at a football game. After the game, the cheerleaders wanted to go to Burger King, but that meant we boys had to change our uniforms while the football players were changing. There was no way I would change in a locker room full of footballers."

"Oh, I would have," Jason laughed sounding like Snidely Whiplash.

I leaned in his direction, "You sound like Snidely Whiplash, Jason."

"Thank you."

"Anytime."

Chris continued, "Back in high school, I knew I was different. I had crushes on some boys, but back then being gay was not allowed in high school. You could be shunned."

"I used to think I'd outgrow being attracted to boys," Neil chuckled.

Suddenly, I heard myself, "Well, that's a really good point, Neil, about not growing out of it. Did you guys ever read Michel Foucault's book?"

"No."

"*The History of Sexuality*?"

"No."

"There are four volumes. I only read the skinny one," I responded.

"We're interested," Jason interjected.

"Okay." I looked around for confirmation.

"Yeah, go ahead," Chris chimed in.

"According to Foucault or at least my interpretation, in early Greece and Rome there wasn't a stigma attached to same sex desire. If a man desired another man, it was considered socially acceptable. Some men really took advantage of this and they created events called symposiums. These were 'men only' parties. I mean men were with other men." Everyone was listening, so I kept going, "These parties still exist, except in our culture, in our society, they're not as public. In ancient Greece and Rome, sexuality wasn't influenced by religious norms; there was no moral issue. This worked well in their society because a man had to marry a virgin. So, prior to marriage, young men had sex with men. It was important for a man to marry a virgin because it ensured a family's financial inheritance would stay in the family, in the familial blood line. But, to your point, Neil, even in ancient Greece, it was expected adolescent boys would 'grow out of it' and eventually desire the virginal woman. But here's the difference, if the male didn't 'grow out of it,' if he didn't desire women, there was no cultural condemnation. No social stigma."

I looked around, "I'm done."

"Well, that's a fine 'how do you do.' We missed out on that, for sure. I do like that explanation," Fernando chuckled.

"Me too!" Chris' curls started doing a sort of do-si-do, square-dance thing with curls passing over each other, hair over hair.

"It would have been so freeing if there was no prejudice. If we were 'allowed' to be gay without suffering rejection or criticism," Thomas interjected.

"Correct, and how about not being taunted at recess," Fernando lamented.

"I know, right?" Thomas affirmed. "How many years do we pretend we're straight, so we don't disappoint people."

Neil responded, "Most of our lives. Hey, I want to read that book."

"The skinny one?"

"Yeah, the skinny one. Anyone want to come with me? Let's meet tomorrow around 5:00, Barnes & Noble on 18th Street."

"Wait, I want to hear the rest of Chris' story," Fernando cajoled.

Chris acknowledged the encouragement. "Where was I? Oh, yeah, 'being gay.' I knew I wouldn't grow out of it, but in high school the best way to hide a guy-crush was to date a girl."

Thomas chuckled, "Not unheard of in my family. Dating girls was a good cover for being gay."

"Yeah, well, this girl in my class, way back in seventh grade, she liked me and back then everyone at school was pairing up. Basically, that meant everyone just held hands and sat together during lunch." A couple of the guys were nodding and mumbling agreement.

"We kept 'dating' for years and then when we were both freshmen, we went out for cheerleading together. It was her suggestion. I probably wanted to cheerlead more than she did, though."

"There were two other guys already on the team. I mean there had to be at least two or you couldn't throw the girls in the air. I guess you could throw them up, but it took two guys to catch 'em on the way down. At this point, Josey and I broke up, or better put, stopped holding hands. We went different ways in high school. She started dating a guy who was on the football team. A real popular guy. Then, in our senior year, she was crowned Homecoming Queen."

"I'll bet that ticked you off, Chris. Did she share the tiara?" Matthew teased.

"Ha, ha. I had my own," Chris chuckled ironically, then sighed. His mood shifted as he leaned back on the folding chair, "Actually, high school was the beginning of a lot of changes."

"What happened?" Neil asked. Everyone in the room seemed engrossed, as though watching a Montgomery Cliff movie.

"Ah, well, in the beginning of our junior year, a new kid transferred to our school and got on the cheerleading team. He was already 'out.' 'Out' to himself, I mean. Nobody would ever have guessed he was gay. It made me think I could 'come out.' It didn't need to be public. Anyway, Morgan was great and when no one was looking we flirted."

Matthew's forehead wrinkled, "What happened to Josephine?"

"She got pregnant. Anyway, Morgan and I kept up the pretense of being straight and we made it all the through our senior year."

"Everything was great until the end of that year. The seniors, our class had a bonfire graduation party. That was normal for the school to do. After that we had our own private graduation parties. It was tradition for the guys to go to the creek and skinny dip. There was a special place where we'd jump off the rocks. It was deep enough. Almost every one of us was drunk, I mean *very* drunk. That didn't matter though and we started jumping off the rocks into the creek."

Chris' tone changed, "Well, Morgan decided to dive off the cliff, not jump like everyone else, he wanted to dive. The creek was deep enough, so you could dive, but we never did. Up till then, I never saw anybody dive."

Chris slid his hand over his forehead, "Morgan dove in. He must have gone out too far or too deep. After a couple of minutes, we thought he was messing with us, pretending to not come up for air. Then we started worrying. Where the hell was he? We flipped out. A bunch of us jumped into the creek, searching, diving down, trying to find him." Chris' gaze slowly moved to the ceiling, as though looking up from the creek bottom. "Nothing." He paused, "Then a couple of guys ran to the nearest house, about a mile away. They called the cops. The cops came and they got in the water trying to find Morgan. Nobody went home that night. Not us, not the cops."

Chris' voice broke, "They dredged the creek in the morning. They found him. Morgan was stuck under a big rock the other side of the creek. He dove too far out, all the way to the other side of the creek. They said it looked like he was trying to come up, trying to surface, but hit his head. It was dark. If it'd been daylight, he might have found the surface. He was under a rock, a ledge."

Chris' head shook, "It was graduation night. Morgan got into Yale. The only kid from school to get accepted there."

Quietly, Thomas asked, "When did this happen?"

"A very long time ago. Six years."

A shiver slid down my spine. If Morgan had lived, would he be in an AIDS group waiting to die?

Chapter 22
The Parent Trap

A second after I sat down, we all heard Richard's voice booming from the hallway, "That was a reunion from hell!" There he was, all smiles, sort of bouncing into the room. Richard had a way with gravity. "If ever again I tell you I'm going to a family reunion, chain me to the radiator."

'That'd be interesting.' I didn't say that.

A few minutes later, Chris arrived breathless. "Hey, welcome back, Richard. Where've you been?"

"At a family reunion and you're just in time to hear all about it."

"Why, what happened?" Chris encouraged Richard to elaborate which was easy to do.

Richard leaned forward tilting his folding chair, then with enthusiasm began, "We've had these reunions before, but this was the first one since I've been diagnosed. Well, leave it to my mother to tell the family that I have AIDS. I told her not to tell them and I've got to give her credit, she pretended she didn't tell them until it was so blatant, she confessed."

"My mother left early to help set up for the reunion. My uncle picked her up. Now, when I get there, I can see all my cousins and aunts, uncles, you name it, everyone's spouse is there, and I'm happy to be there. I see my favorite aunt, so I start waving. She isn't waving back. Maybe she can't see it's me or whatever, so I start walking over to her for a hug. She backs away and nearly falls off the picnic bench. Then her wine goes all over her and she looks at me, as though it's my fault she spilled her wine. Like a bat out of hell, she races into the house yelling, 'Don't do that again, Richard.' Right! Like I spilled her red wine when I'm six feet away and purposely did it on purpose. Well, her yelling at me certainly announced my presence and everyone stopped talking and looked at me as though I spilled an entire vineyard of wine on my aunt. Some of them really look upset, like 'what-the-hell-are-you-doing-here.' Not everybody, but just about."

"At this point, my relatives start acting like I'm not there, ignoring me. Here's a good one, across the lawn, my mother's brother comes up to me and says, 'You use these paper plates, not those.' Then he says, 'my garbage goes in a particular bag,' which my uncle holds up. It got my name on it. The bag has a 'Richard's garbage' sign, which is also what I'm starting to feel like. Keep in mind, I still haven't said anything yet, not a word and I'm thinking I've been here less than five/ten minutes and so far, I've been yelled at by my aunt, my uncle insinuates I'm garbage and my mother snitched on me."

"Jesus, you weren't prepared for that reception. You were blindsided," Thomas interjected.

"Right! It turns out, my mother told them. She told *everyone* at the reunion I have AIDS. Now that I'm thinking about it, I'll bet she told people who weren't at the reunion.

I specifically told her not to tell anyone. But no, she told *everyone*. At this point, my aunt is still freaking out in a wine-dyed t-shirt, my uncle's guarding the family garbage pail from getting AIDS, and my mother's broadcasting my situation to all of Florida. I start looking around at everyone and I'm hoping it's just the old people who are flipped out because they don't read up on AIDS and haven't a clue that I'm not going to infect them. They probably think they'll catch AIDS if I sit on the picnic bench or if they walk too close to my paper plates."

"I keep looking around and I see my cousin, my favorite cousin, Jeff, who's around my age. We played together as kids. It was Jeff who introduced me to the joys of being gay when I was nine years old or maybe it was a mutual introduction. Yeah, it was mutual, but when he got married, he let me know he's not gay. He also said *I* touched *him*. Whatever. Jeff is sitting at another table and looks like he'd seen a ghost when he spots me. I wave and he half waved like 'stay where you are and pretend we don't know each other' wave. I felt like yelling, 'Hey, Jeff, I didn't give you AIDS when we were nine!"

"Richard, how come you didn't leave?" Neil's curiosity peaked, loudly.

"I was hungry! I'd come a long way and I wasn't going to let them push me out of a reunion. A family reunion that I belong to. Forget that!"

"This gets weird-er. I go over to the food, right? At these reunions, everyone brings a dish and I do too. I make my Phenomenal Portuguese Potatoes. My mother says she's going to take the potatoes to the reunion because she's going early. My uncle comes to pick her up, but he stays in the car, which is unusual. I know she's got vision problems, so my uncle drives her when she needs to get somewhere."

"Wait, I've gone astray. Let me get back to the reunion. No one is talking to me, so I may as well eat. I start loading up my plate. Some of them are watching me, upset, like I'm around the food and now the coleslaw has AIDS. What the hell! They think the virus is leaking through the plastic spoons that I'm relegated to use, like I'm poisoning the stuff on the table, through the spoon?"

Richard's anger increased, "Finally, my cousin, Sara, comes over, puts her arm around me and wants me to sit with her. Of course, Sara apologizes for them, and tries to make me feel better, but at this point, I'm angry. Should I leave? No, I'm hungry. Now I realize my uncle left early, so I have to stay to drive my mother home, which means I have to stay for the entire time. Poor Sara is stuck with me for the duration of the reunion. Who knows, they probably think she's infected now, too. Maybe not, because she's not a gay man and this is a gay man disease. My relatives probably think AIDS is gender specific. Finally, the reunion is over. Nobody ate my Phenomenal Portuguese Potatoes because apparently potatoes have AIDS-by-association. I'm really upset and when my mother and I are in the car, I said, 'Why did you tell them I have AIDS? I told you not to. I told you. I didn't *ask* you. I *told* you."

"'Oh, Richard,' she says. 'I need support from the family. These people are my family. Of course, I told them. I need people to talk to.'"

Richard slapped his knees, "I was furious! Every one of them? You talked to all of them?"

"She says, 'I told everyone so no one would feel left out.'" Richard's hands shot into the air, "I couldn't believe it. You? *You* need support? I've got AIDS and you need support? Then she says, 'Now Richard, you're not the only person this AIDS thing affects. Don't you think I'm hurt, too? I'm a mother of a boy with AIDS.'"

Richard nearly catapulted out of his chair, "Do you believe she said that? It hurts *her* that I've got AIDS and I'd better be sympathetic to her? What the hell?"

Neil interjected, "Richard, that was supposed to be a fun reunion. You were looking forward to it."

Jason chimed in, "Well, it's like Thomas Wolf says, *You Can't Go Home Again.*"

Thomas sneered, "I agree with that, wholeheartedly."

Chapter 23
Fabrications

A few weeks later, almost at the end of the session Richard sat up straighter, pushed his hair from his eyes, and began, "I have a question about AZT. You remember I told you my T-4 count was below 500."

Richard looked at me, "Do you know we're supposed to have about 1000 of those cells?"

I nodded 'yes,' which was true.

Richard continued, "Initially, my doctor started me on AZT at 1500mg a day."[20]

Fernando chimed in, "Well, that's what I used to take."

"Yeah, me too, but my dose has been lowered," Neil interjected.

"Mine, too," Matthew added as he leaned back on his folding chair. "My father wants me to see our family doctor. I'm not sure why he thinks a local doctor might know something more or different than my doctor here, but it'll make my father feel better, so I'll go."

"He probably wants to feel like he's doing something for you," Chris commented. "Probably hoping there's some other way to fight the virus."

Richard looked around, "You guys ever want to just stop taking this damn drug?"

"Yeah, I want to stop, but I won't," Thomas interjected. Some of the guys mumbled agreement, some didn't.

Richard continued, "My doctor said I'm really anemic, and we all know what that means."[21]

"Yes, we all know about that, and I have more KS lesions," Matthew added. Everyone in the group nodded in agreement.

I was taken aback. Do they *all* have advanced KS? I looked at Jason who slowly nodded, 'yes.'

"We hide them," Jason whispered.

Richard continued, "I'm dizzy all the time now." He looked at Jason, "When you ran the group at the hospital were their symptoms like ours?"

"I don't want to talk about it," Jason retorted.

Richard seemed unphased by Jason's abruptness, "I don't know. I feel exhausted the moment I get up in the morning."

"I totally understand," Fernando commiserated. "It's an effort to stand up. But, let me tell you, no matter where I am, no matter what time it is, I just plain pass out. I'll probably have to start taking pills for narcolepsy."

Thomas added, "I'm glad ACT UP wants the dose lowered. Kudos to Vito."

Chris confessed, "Actually, I'm on a fourth of the dose. My doctor is skeptical about the trial results. This was last week."

"Depending on who your doctor is, determines how much AZT you get," Jason interjected.

"We're guineapigs," Fernando lamented.

Matthew interrupted, "Getting back to my trip home. I'll be here next week but not the following week. I don't know what my father's got planned. I'll stay in touch, though."

"Thanks for reminding me, Matthew," Richard chimed in. "I won't be here for a few weeks. A friend of mine wants me to stay with him. It might be the last time we see each other. So, I'll be in Connecticut for a few weeks. Oh, and my mother wants me to go to Florida, again. I told her I'd visit, but not if there's a reunion. Anyway, that's down the road, but I'll be in Connecticut for a week or two, maybe three."

Matthew grinned, sort of an empty grin, then asked, "Are we done? Are we done for the day?"

"Yes, we're done," I responded, glancing around the room. They were all way too thin. Everyone but Chris was too thin, too gray, and too exhausted.

Chapter 24
Waving Through
a Window Dressing

It was the week before Matthew was to go home. He was late. Matthew typically sat directly across from me. It was nice to look at him because he was often smiling. Not always, but often. Maybe his smile was meant to comfort people around him or meant as protection from his own unwanted emotions. Sometimes he had a big smile, sometimes it was a slight ends-of-mouth upturn. It depended on the topic. Unfortunately, Matthew's grin mutated whatever depth of emotion he felt.

Matthew had chiseled features juxtaposed onto a sweet, adorable face framed by thick light brown hair and matching eyes. He had a perfect body, albeit too thin. Thin was the only weight available to men with full-blown AIDS.

Matthew grew up in Texas, so he had that 'bless your heart' thing right alongside his abiding grin. I'd never met a Texan before, except when I changed planes in Houston. Matthew was from East Texas. I didn't know Texas bothered to make that distinction. East Texas, West Texas. What about the Oklahoma pan handle that used to be Texas?

Northwest Temporary Texas, maybe? I'll bet losing that handle upset the Friendship State.

At the time, the only East and West I knew about was in Manhattan. In New York City, in the late 1980s, the Westside of the island was the most desirable neighborhood for gay men, especially if they opened antique shops. Prior to the influx of gay, the Upper Westside was a mess. Full of squatters, abandoned buildings, graffiti, visible drug sales and frequent late-night gun shots. When the antique shops and gay men came to the Upper Westside, everybody called it gentrification. Gay gentrification areas included Chelsea on the Lower Westside, the Westside of Greenwich Village especially Christopher Street, the Rambles at the Upper Westside of Central Park, the Westside Theater district by Hell's Kitchen, and maybe a little bit of the Garment District in Midtown particularly during Fashion Week which was Matthew's nirvana.

As I mentioned earlier, Matthew was a window dresser for a Fifth Avenue exclusive department store. One of the highlights was when Matthew came to group with little bits of window dressing sparkle in his hair. Anyone who sat next to him had the wonderful option of pulling sequins or various colored common threads out of Matthew's thick wavy hair. It was that kind of never-going-to-recede hairline that made balding bearded guys envious.

In the past, Matthew told us about meeting famous clothing designers. For a while, one of his lovers was a big-shot designer. I'd never heard of Matthew's lover because I usually wore Laura Ashley dresses. Anyway, this big shot designer loaned Matthew some beautiful one-of-a-kind outfits that probably nobody else had the guts to wear in public. Some of Matthew's designer's shirts had space-age pointy shoulder pads that were extremely distracting during group sessions, especially when paired with sparkly fabric remnants in his hair. I believe others in the group, those with a sense of style (like me) were also impressed with Matthew's clothing stardom. He didn't mind getting attention when he wore designer clothing. For example, if a stranger commented on his clothing, he'd say who designed it, then walk away swirling and posing to highlight fashion artistry at its best advantage. I was cool with that.

I remember when Matthew first talked about window dressing. He said, 'no one he worked with knew he had AIDS.' Matthew thought if the girls in the store knew he had AIDS, they would panic and apply for disability. It was interesting, the only people who dreaded going on disability were people with AIDS.

Chapter 25
The Mink Coat

As I mentioned, it was the week before Matthew was to go home. About ten minutes after this week's session began, Matthew swirled through the door wearing a fantastic full-length mink coat. Walking to his chair, he pulled the mink collar tighter, sat down, then snuggling as much as he could into the warmth of mink. He didn't seem to be the least bit interested in taking it off. I wasn't going to question it. Unfortunately, my 'assistant group leader' thought otherwise. "Aren't you hot?" Jason asked, his upper lip curled.

"No. Isn't this a wonderful coat?" Matthew stood up and with a runway-model-turn showed the fine details of the coat.

"It's my mother's coat." He looked at Jason, "I'm loving being in my mother's beautiful mink coat." Matthew's smile shook his head as he sat down. "Her coat keeps me toasty warm. Since I started AZT, I'm cold a lot of the time. So, Mom sent me her coat."

"I forgot. When were you get diagnosed?" Jason asked.
"In '86."
"Me, too."

"You and I were probably hospitalized around the same time with PCP, with pneumonia."

Jason nodded agreement, "It all starts with PCP."

"Anyway," Matthew continued. "I saw my doctor again yesterday. I decided to see him before I met with our family doctor. My CD4 count plummeted which of course means my immune system sucks. He wants me to stay on the lower dose of AZT."[22]

Chris slid in, "A lot of people are doing a little better on it."

"I'm good on the lower dose," Thomas added.

Jason interjected, "Doctors don't have a clue about the right AZT dose. Nobody does."

"Nor do they don't know the outcome of the dose," Neil's sarcasm peaked.

"I can't stand these KS lesions. I got a few more since last week." Fernando shifted in his chair, unbuttoned his collar, and pointed to a reddish blue/black scab. "I got them injected on Monday."

"I get them injected, too," Matthew lamented.

"Are yours multiplying? Are they getting bigger?" Fernando asked.

"Mine are, definitely." Thomas threw in his two cents.

"Both. It's so weird, you know. Doctors wait until the scabs are really bad before they inject them. I don't know if they have a standard chart for 'bad-enough.' Who created the chart and who determines what's bad, or what's over-bad?"

Matthew rolled his eyes, "It's like in the morning, I look at them and think, I can't wait till these get really bad so I can get them injected."

Fernando shifted in agreement, "I don't know why we have to wait until they became florid."

"I'm with you there," Jason announced.

Fernando inhaled exasperation, "You know, I tried to get into the trials, but they wouldn't take me. I already had OIs."[23] Fernando shook his head, "So far they haven't showed up on my face."

"Well, even with injections, they come back," Thomas added.

Fernando continued, "A friend of mine has them on his face. He told me people grimace or look away. I don't blame 'em. Who wants to see KS? My friend said nobody gets physically close to him. I understand that. I've felt the same way. I won't take off my shirt unless it's for the doctor, not even for the nurse."

"Yeah, when people see KS, my friend said they react like he has leprosy. As if they'll catch it by looking at him." Ferando's face stiffened, "It doesn't matter, though. There's no time."

At first, it was difficult to discern if Fernando was shutting down emotionally or wanting to open the flood gate. Okay, it was the flood gate. Tears fell at will. Soon Fernando's face became streaked. He wiped his eyes on his sleeve unknowingly exposing a scab barely above his wrist.

Instead of covering it, "Oh, I know, another scab."

"No, it's the streaks. You have red streaks on you face," Neil responded.

Fernando shrugged, "I'm allergic to my tears. Sort of insult to injury, isn't it? Every part of me is melting." He grinned sardonically, "How ironic, I can't even cry right."

Matthew's seat was next to Fernando. "Are you okay, Fernando?" He moved closer and in almost slow motion put his arm around Fernando and whispered, "Hey, you're in good company."

Fernando was barely audible, "You're the first person who's held me in a long time and in mink, no less."

"You should have asked me sooner," Matthew tenderly quipped. "How about I walk you home tonight?"

"I'll walk with you, too. I go in the same direction," Neil added.

Jason took a deep breath and without ceremony, "Let's end for today. It's almost time anyway."

Matthew hastily interrupted, "Oh, wait! I won't be here next week, remember I mentioned last week?"

Suddenly, Matthew plopped back to his seat leaving him to re-wrap his mother's mink. "I didn't tell you guys. I spoke to my father again and apparently, he didn't tell me the first time we talked, but another reason he wants me home, besides my going to another doctor is that my mother was just diagnosed with lung cancer."

No one said, 'maybe she'll recover.' They didn't ask for details. Not many people survived lung cancer in the 1980s.

Chapter 26
St. Bartholomew

The AIDS virus was incredibly duplicitous. During the first year I ran the group, it wore a Janus mask, sometimes hiding symptoms often duping its host. In the 1980s, many people held hope that AZT would fight the virus and provide additional time. But what kind of additional time?

Now, what was once hidden under clothing became increasingly difficult to mask, weight loss, KS, and the ravages of AZT. Initially, AZT appeared to slow down the virus. But how much AZT? Too much, you die. Too little, you die. No AZT, you die. The AZT trials produced incomplete and biased results.[24] Did the public know that? Did they even care?

This might sound off point, but the AIDS epidemic reminded me of the Huguenot victims in Massey, France, in 1572. Just when the French Protestants began feeling accepted in a Catholic country and no longer needed to hide their beliefs, they were brutally killed in the Saint Bartholomew Massacre. My men were born during a time when being gay was marginally accepted. It wasn't until the 1960s that the tide began to turn. Now, in 1988, they are dying. Every day became a Saint Bartholomew Massacre.

It was the holiday season, 1989/1990. Now, whenever I entered the session room, there were empty folding chairs. Vito's chair was frequently empty because he lectured, taught, and ACT'ed Up. Matthew had been absent for a while due to his mother's cancer. Thomas' chair was newly empty. Jason said Thomas' sister was visiting during the holidays and he'd a few miss sessions until she left. Richard was either in Connecticut or Florida. Fernando had been hospitalized, according to his newly hired caretaker. She also said he was better and couldn't wait to return to group.

This was our first meeting after the two-week Christmas/New Year holiday, 1990.

"Let's begin," the chair next to me said. At this point, I was used to Jason. He turned to me, "I have an update on Thomas. His sister contacted me over the holiday. Apparently, she wasn't just here to visit. Thomas is in the hospital, and he asked for her help. We visited him New Year's Day, in the hospital."

"How is he?"

"He's not good."

"We asked his sister to call you."

"She didn't. This is the first I'm hearing it."

"Well," Jason continued. "He's in not-so-good shape. His T-3 cell count was way low. He fell asleep while we were visiting, so we just hung out in his room for a while. He woke up a couple of times, talked to us and then fell back to sleep. We left after a while."

"Hold on a minute, Jason," Chris interjected. "You're leaving out a very important piece."

"That's okay," Jason resisted.

Chris persisted, "That's not fair, tell her what happened."

"You tell her what happened," Jason challenged.

"Okay, great!" Chris began, "We're all getting ready to leave when we see Jason lean over Thomas' face, almost nose to nose."

Jason reacted, "Yeah, I was furious."

Chris continued, "That's for sure. So, Jason is in Thomas' face and all of a sudden Jason yells, 'I'm not through with you. You better not die.' We're all stunned, but not as stunned as Thomas." Chris shot a look at Jason. "I'm surprised you didn't give him a heart attack. I mean, Jason can be very loud. So, here comes the nurse. The whole hospital must have heard him. The nurse storms in and Jason is still leaning over Thomas' face. Then the nurse yells, 'You all get out. Right now. Leave.'"

Jason smiled with a Cheshire cat grin, "Yeah, that's what I did."

Chris continued, "You won't believe this." He looked at everyone then back to me, "Thomas was discharged on Monday. He'll be here. He'll be here next week. Sometimes it's good to yell at people."

"You bet, Jason," Neil emphatically agreed.

I leaned back on my chair and kept listening. There they were, each one of them telling various versions of the 'Jason nose to nose with Thomas story.' It was quite impressive.

Apparently, Jason was right. No one in this group is allowed to die.

Chapter 27
Coda

I arrived early to GMHC that evening. Everyone was seated, waiting.

"Am I late?"

"I've got good news and bad news," Jason announced.

"Fernando is on the mend."

"The bad news?"

"The bad news is horrible. Thomas' sister called. He passed a few days after the hospital discharged him. His funeral will be at the Metropolitan Community Church of New York. We're all going to meet there."

"Everyone in the group knows?"

"Yes."

"Do you want me to attend?"

"No. We need you here."

"Get this," Jason added. "Thomas' father wants the coroner's report to say it was kidney failure. Thomas died from the virus, not kidney failure. His father doesn't want people to know why he died." Jason's tone turned bitter, "How ironic, Thomas. Once again you disappointed your father. Even in death, his father resented him."

I was stunned, "I need a moment to recover."

Jason nodded, "Sure."

Neil interrupted, "I had dinner with Richard over the weekend. Correction, I ate dinner, Richard was too nauseous to eat. He didn't look good. He's going to Florida to stay with his mother for a few weeks." Neil coughed, then cleared his throat, "I have a feeling he won't return."

Neil was right. Richard never returned.

Jason cleared his throat, "I think we should talk about getting new members. We should add some new guys."

"Do you want to talk about losing Thomas, or Richard?"

"No." My proposal was unanimously declined.

"We need to talk about adding new members," Jason quickly added.

"New members will change the group dynamics, which is not necessarily a bad development," I interjected. "If this group is going to continue, we will need new members. Do any of you disagree. It's your group and you decide."

I was hoping that if the group continued, the pledge to not die continued.

"What do you mean? What group dynamics?" Chris questioned.

"You've been together for a while. You know each other. New people will alter these relationships," I explained.

Neil questioned, "What if we don't like them?"

Chris retorted, "What if they don't like us?"

"How could they not like us?" Jason scanned the room. "If you don't want new people, I'll go along with the group."

"No, I think Jason has a point," Neil chimed in. "New members might make it easier for us. We'll be seeing people and not empty chairs."

"Like I said," Jason reiterated. "I'll go along with the group." Abruptly he turned to me, "Do you want new people?" I stared at him. 'Oh yeah, right,' I'm thinking. I'm not treading on that minefield. If they like the new guys, fine, but what if they feel dethroned. What if they *don't* like the new guys. I might get blamed for choosing the wrong new guys. I agreed with myself to not answer Jason's question, so I sidetracked it.

"I think there are valid reasons for adding new people. There will be new ingredients in the mix. It might not feel comfortable at first. That's not the right word. It'll be an adjustment." I scanned their faces. "Never mind." I corrected myself, "You guys are experts at adjusting. But I'm wondering what it will be like for you to tell the new guys about yourselves." I paused, "About what's happened in the group. Losing Thomas, losing Richard."

A couple of the guys shifted on their folding chair. "On the other hand, maybe it'll be similar to the dynamics of your early meetings. Who has what role, how will you relate, will the group remain cohesive or feel penetrated. Adding new people might be a spanner in the works. Who knows."

Chris' face tilted, "I thought it was *A Spaniard in the Works*."

"No, that was John Lennon," I retorted. "Shall we do this? If so, how many guys do you want?"

Neil reacted, "Two."

"I agree," Chris seconded the motion.

Jason looked at me, "Just two."

"I've got it. Two."

The next day I called GMHC.

"I'd like to interview two potential new members for my group."

"You should interview four."

"They only want two."

"I'll set up four, anyway. Just in case."

"I only need two."

"You might change your mind."

"The guys want two. They want to keep the group homogenous. No IV drug users. Just gay men."

"Not a problem, four guys, no IV drug users. I'll set up the interviews. You're interviewing four gay men."

"I'm only taking two."

"It's a good idea to interview four."

I interviewed four men at GMHC. I choose two because that administrator wasn't going to tell me how to live my life. One fellow was named David, who pronounced his name Da-veed. The other guy was named Raul, so there was no problem there. I told them both they could join the group the end of the month.

During the interview, Da-veed gently announced, "You'd better let them know Da-veed is coming." The other one, Raul didn't say anything regarding dramatic foreshadowing.

I left the interviews at GMHC and hung out until time to begin the group.

An aside: Thinking back to 1988 when the group started, the men had symptoms that weren't visible. In 1989, their symptoms were more obvious, and their hospitalizations more frequent. By 1990, my group members knew their bodies, their time, and their lives were ending. Within these two years, most of the public thought AZT might be the magic pill, a savior medication, a drug that could provide time until a cure was found. It's amazing how so many of us were duped,[25] and how many gay men remained hopeful-enough to add two more members.

Chapter 28
February 1990

A week or so later, the group session began when Jason announced, "You're not going to believe this, but Fernando's coming this evening." He looked at me, "Do you know he's coming." I shook my head, 'yes.'

"Jason, you're serious?" Chris responded full of excitement.

"Yes. His caretaker called saying he would be here tonight," Jason confirmed.

"Wonderful!" Chris exclaimed. The mood in the group was immediately elevated. It was lovely sitting, chatting, waiting for Fernando.

Five minutes passed, then ten minutes. Jason seemed unusually anxious, "Maybe Fernando's health changed since I spoke to his caretaker, but she assured me he would be here." We all snuck glances at the doorway until we heard voices echo in the hallway.

"It's Fernando!" Chris announced. We could hear him giving his caretaker navigational directions. Then, within a second, there they were: Fernando, Fernando's caretaker, Fernando's wheelchair, and Fernando's cane carefully placed across his lap.

A few of the guys started standing up to help, but Fernando's caretaker waved her finger 'no' having been forewarned he did not want to appear helpless. She locked the wheels as Fernando gripped the handles, elbows raised like an egret's wings before flight. The longer Fernando remained in the doorway, the longer we studied him. How is it possible that he's even thinner than before?

Ferando was barely a shadow of his former self. I attempted to avert my gaze, but we were all stuck in stare. How could this happen in such a short amount of time? He had been thin, yes, but now he was skin on bones. He barely resembled himself. Fernando's caretaker removed his goose-down coat revealing a flannel shirt that overwhelmed his upper body. His blue jeans seemed entirely empty. When he took off his wool cap, his hair loss was evident.

"I know, I lost my hair." Smiling, Fernando joked, "I made a trade with my doctor. He gave me some pills that made my hair fall out and in return, I paid his bill." Most of us smiled, using opportunity to gather short-lived composure.

"Are you sure you don't need help?" Chris lamented. Chris' body seemed ready to bolt off his folding chair. One leg was under the seat and the other bent in runner's formation.

"No, no," Fernando shook his hand warding off Chris. "I'm fine." He signaled his caretaker to lock the wheelchair that she'd already locked, and announced, "I'd liked to walk on my own."

His caretaker hesitated; already aware his shame overpowered his body. He wanted to appear as healthy as the others. What an oxymoron.

Again, Fernando pushed down on the handles struggling to stand. Slowly, he achieved a bent over stance, then in trying to straighten, began to sway. He turned, indicating his need for help. She held his arm, deeply indenting his flannel shirt. When he no longer swayed, she let go. Fernando lifted his head as his bent over stance morphed into a shaky but standing body. He looked at us and with a surprised smile said, "Hey, you guys. I made it!" Fernando was joyful, standing, and scared stiff. His smile masked grimaces of extreme pain as he took his first two shuffled steps. He stopped, swayed just a little bit, pivoted toward the caretaker, "I'll take my cane."

"Good." She looked apprehensive perhaps deciding between help and shame vs her job duties. Grasping the cane, Fernando's fingers slowly looped the handle creating movement similar to a dowsing stick. Another shuffled step entered the room. Fernando gave a backward goodbye-wave to his wheelchair indicating its removal with his caretaker. Fortunately, both wheelchair and caretaker ignored his directive and remained on alert a few minutes longer.

It was obvious Fernando's pain increased with each step. Again, he swayed, stopped then re-steadied himself. I held my breath. We all did. He deliberately bit his lip perhaps confusing location of pain. With each step, my thoughts banged from one side of my brain to the other in rhythm with his shuffle. I tried to bargain, "It's too soon. You're breaking your pledge, Fernando. No one dies in this group." My mind felt pummeled under a deluge of partial thoughts ending with an elongated 'Noooooooo.'

Chris stood up and with intent, announced, "One day you're going to help me, so I'm paying forward. Don't complain. You'll hurt my feelings if you don't let me help. You'd do the same for me." Fernando's shame softened as Chris slid his arm around him, "You don't need to worry, Miss Scarlett," Chris' voice lilted. Fernando forced another smile. Then, deadpan announced, "Actually, I feel more like Miss Mellie. No, Miss Pittypat."

"Well then," Chris laughed. "I'm here to let you know the knife is under the bed to cut the pain. At your service, Miss Pittypat."

Neil quipped, "Why did you pick Miss Pittypat? I would have chosen Scarlet."

"When you need help, we'll do Scarlet," Chris joked.

Slowly, Fernando and Chris matched shuffle to step accompanied by cane thumps on concrete floor. It was as though Fernando's cane announced his presence, his pace, and his illness. Perhaps Chris wanted to drown out each thump because his voice grew louder quoting moments from *Gone with the Wind*. This painful yet sweet scene felt unreal, paradoxical, cognitively dissonant. How could this have happened so fast? Good lord! I'm watching him die. Stay in the moment, I reprimanded my mind as it stuttered, stammered, and juxtaposed faces of each man.

Fernando gave a sigh of relief as Chris lowered him onto the metal folding chair. "Well, I think I'm almost done with all this."

"What do you mean *done with all this*?" Jason was a master of confrontation.

Fernando nodded preparing to speak, "I can hardly eat real food; you know what I mean? I've got an intestinal infection and I can't digest. I've been on an intravenous drip. When I was in the hospital, they hooked a drip into the side of my stomach. It got a landslide of Ensure. This drip thing fed me all day long and let me tell you, the claim that Ensure tastes good, well, I wouldn't know."

I glanced around. Did they feel as scared as I felt? What am I doing here? They'll all start looking like this. One at a time. I can't do this. I just can't watch them die.

"The intravenous line keeps getting infected and then, bang, I end up back in the hospital." Fernando's frustration peaked, "Apparently, I'm so anemic, I'm pathetic, absolutely pathetic. I'm pathetically anemic." His fingers folded as though giving up or maybe in prayer.

I can't recall what else happened in this session. I've tried to remember, but nothing returns memory other than feelings of desperation.

After what seemed like forever, someone said, "I'll see you next week. Session is over." The guys straggled out. Someone fetched Fernando's caretaker and wheelchair.

Jason, however, remained seated next to me. "This will get worse!" he warned. "You know this will get a lot worse." He stood up, maybe debating if he should tell me how worse it will get. Shaking his head, he left. I listened to his footsteps until they faded. I lost track of time until I heard the janitor's rattling buckets, "Is everybody out?"

"No, I'm still here. It's just me."

"I'm locking up!" the janitor yelled.

"I'm leaving. I'm leaving." I grabbed my blue swing coat and tried to focus on getting out of the building. Focusing failed. I bumped into the hallway wall and the wall retaliated by bouncing me off the other one. I felt like

Tommy the Blind Pinball Wizard's silver pinball that *The Who* metaphorically sang about.[26]

Chapter 29
March 1990

Although Fernando was physically stressed at our last meeting, we knew he was determined to make this week's session. Entering the room, he was smiling to beat the band, or perhaps smiling for the boys in *his* band. I watched him struggle to stand up, say goodbye to his caretaker and wheelchair, and let Chris help him walk to his hard gray folding chair. Last week he said he'd lost well over twenty pounds. Weight loss was standard for people infected with AIDS, but Fernando's weight loss was frightening.

Up until recently, I must have been steeped in so much denial, I hadn't seen the extent of Fernando's symptoms. In addition to being thinner, his skin tone looked dusty; a grayish hue that made the hollow below his cheekbones more pronounced. The area between his upper lip and nose was sunken, as though muscle melted. Chris helped him sit down. All body parts seemed dependent on help from others. I found myself staring at him. Shivers ran through my body. If Chris holds this fragile Fernando too tightly, will he shatter?

Once again, Fernando's presence created a buzz, but it soon stalled. Neil looked worried, "Hey Fernando, what's up? What's the update?"

Fernando sighed, "I'm so relieved to be here." Versions of 'so are we' came from everyone.

"I'm happy you're here two weeks in a row. You're on a winning streak," I said faking reality.

"It's been eventful, that's for sure. So much has happened since last week." Fernando's smile was fading. "I'll tell the events chronically, otherwise, I'll get lost. My memory isn't what it used to be." He leaned back, sighed, and began, "Matthew and I have stayed in touch, especially when I was hospitalized because he got hospitalized around the same time. We've been on a similar health/medical path. If he got sick, I'd come down with something, too. We seemed to share the pace of illnesses. You probably don't remember; we were diagnosed around the same time. Matthew and I joked that his health might foretell mine and vice versa."

Fernando's mood was visibly slipping, "We were both hospitalized around the same time." Fernando was repeating himself, but nobody cared if he said the same thing all session long, as long as he was with us. AIDS could fill memory with potholes.

He tried to smile, but failed, "Did Matthew contact you when his mom died?"

"No," Jason and I responded in unison.

Jason added, "As far as I know, he hasn't been in touch with anyone here."

Chris interjected, "I figured he was overwhelmed taking care of his mother's health. It made sense that he'd be out of touch."

"I called him a lot," Fernando recounted. "Especially after his mom passed. Matthew really struggled with her death. Whenever I called, his father answered the phone. I chatted with his father until Matthew got to the phone." Fernando attempted a faint grin, "Every time Matthew and I talked, it would be for a long while. When we hung up neither of us had an ounce of saliva. Mostly we talked about his health, my health, his meds or mine. You remember, Matthew's father wanted him to see their local doctor. Well, the doctor convinced Matthew to increase his AZT dose."

Fernando's voice dramatically rose, "Matthew's new dose seemed to work for a little while."

"He had a preexisting OIs, right?" Jason asked.

"Yeah, he did. We were the same when it came to our white blood cell count. You know, this new level of AZT made Matthew dizzier than usual. More headachy and nauseas." Fernando sat straighter, perhaps adjusting his own nausea. "Matthew said he was incredibly anemic and weak and because of our past similarity of symptom, I thought we were experiencing the same level, but that wasn't true. Matthew complained about getting a horrible head rush whenever he stood up. He said the room would spin and he feared falling down." Fernando lowered his head cupping it with both hands, "Actually, Matthew was passing out according to his dad. His white blood cell count must have been way lower than mine, but he never said that." Fernando's mind stumbled, "Did I tell you this chronologically?" Fernando stared into space so we waited for him.

In a barely audible voice, as though whispering to himself, "It must have been *way lower*." Fernando's face reddened, "Last week, it was last week that Matthew passed."

The room echoed a silent solidarity. Everyone was staring at nothing, just like Fernando. He started rocking side to side. His face reddened, then paled, "You guys, I'm in much better shape than him. I mean, I got out of the hospital." I tried to catch my breath, but it felt like inhaling a street sign on a miserable journey. Fernando tried to clear his throat but attempts to speak choked him.

"The wake is tomorrow. Matthew's father is arranging it. I mean it's already arranged." Shaking his head, "First, Matthew's father buried his wife and now, his son." Fernando's shoulders sank as tears flowed into canals for more tears.

The remainder of the session focused on Matthew's death, on Thomas's death, on Fernando's return, on AZT, AIDS, and OIs. Finally, the session was over. The guys negotiated who would help Fernando. Neil took his left arm while Chris slipped Fernando's coat over his shoulders. All three seemed to express Fernando's weakness with each step toward his wheelchair and caretaker. Soon all my men were all gone.

My eyes felt sore and blurry from tears kept hostage. A few escaped gathering my belongings. I turned out the light. Then, almost mechanically, I looked into the dark empty room. Fernando is next.

Chapter 30
The Trouble with Taxis

Fernando is next. The thought swirled in my mind as I left GMHC that evening. Outside, the wind nearly knocked me over and prolonged each step onto the sidewalk. My blue swing coat had a Michelin doughboy look as wind ballooned it from hem upward. Finally arriving at the corner, I began the fruitless endeavor of hailing a taxi in freezing weather concurrently struggling with the loop in my mind, 'I can't live through each of their deaths. I don't want to see them suffer. I don't want to watch them die.'

I didn't *see* Matthew's health deteriorating, nor did I *see* Thomas' last weeks of life. Jason and Chris' health seemed 'alright,' so far. I had *seen* Richard's weight dropping. Neil was losing weight, as well, but still mobile. Yes, everyone's KS was more visible. But this was different, Fernando was quickly diminishing in front of my eyes.

The taxi arrived. I was so distracted, I closed the door on the hem of my enormous blue swing coat. Now, I was immobilized in the back seat of the taxi, physically and emotionally.

"Where to, lady?"

"88th and Central Park West." The taxi began moving. The first neighborhood we drove through was Chelsea, a very gay area. There were men holding hands, eating together in restaurants. Some were dressed to the nines out on dates, some wearing suits returning home from work. They looked healthy. It was me who felt unwell. Then, I thought, "If I'm not 'well,' I shouldn't be involved with GMHC. It's not fair to the group. I should quit. Yes, absolutely, I need to quit. I'm not really needed at GMHC." I comforted myself with, 'there are lots of therapists who want to lead groups at GMHC.' I would be replaced, quickly replaced. I'll tell Jason he can take over. I'll quit as soon as possible. What a relief. I'm done.

My thoughts raced as the taxi driver hit every red light on 8th Avenue providing a ton of time to ruminate. I decided the red traffic lights were signs that mercury was in retrograde. Mercury was telling me to leave the group. Honestly, I don't understand Mercury. What direction is retrograde and who decided which way went where?

Chapter 31
The Rain is Tess, The Fire's Jo, and They Call the Wind Mariah

The taxi was probably around Lincoln Center when my rumination gave way to tears. I cried until the taxi reached my apartment building. I cried in the elevator, in the hallway, entering my apartment, and preparing for bed. I laid down but couldn't sleep. The next morning brought no relief, just more rumination. "I can't do it. I'm quitting. I'll tell my supervisor. She'll agree. Then I'll tell GMHC." I decided to convince myself and add various justifications. "Look this is clear to me," I told myself. "I have to quit because my private patients take priority, and what about my home life, and Jason is definitely able to lead the group."

It's not unusual for recently graduated psychoanalysts to remain in supervision a few years after analytic training. I couldn't wait to tell my supervisor I was quitting GMHC. I figured even if she didn't initially agree, she had to realize it was the best thing for me, and of course, (I concocted a fantastic rationale) it was the best thing for the group. My supervisor's office was on Central Park West in the El

Dorado, three blocks from my apartment which is enough time to resume crying enroute.

In New York, crying as you walk down the street means you've just left your therapist's office, or your boyfriend is a jerk. There's no social stigma. In addition, I was hoping all this crying would dehydrate me so I wouldn't cry in front of my supervisor and she could continue to think I was an adult. As soon as I sat down in her office, I felt pathetic. Finally, I teared out an extremely important question, "How come I'm not dehydrated?" She looked quizzical and didn't answer. "Listen, I just can't do this anymore. I have to quit the AIDS group and GMHC." Within a second, her head shook in that 'no' direction. Desperate, I pleaded, "It's destroying me. I'm not sleeping, I don't have an appetite, and I'm afraid this will affect my private practice." She wasn't convinced. So I told her, "I can't jeopardize my private practice and the guys in my group are fine on their own and it's important to let Jason run the group to increase his level of self-esteem." Of course, Jason had plenty of self-esteem, but I was on a roll and guilt often works on people/my supervisor.

"You can't stop. You can't stop until they stop." My voice pitched, "Well, I don't want to *be there* when they stop. You don't know what this is turning into. I can't keep losing them. They're dying. Look, if I keep this up, I'll be a basket case."

"You can't quit."

I had no idea my voice could hit an operatic untrained soprano level, "It's wrong for me to lead the group solo. I cannot do it. It will destroy me."

All I needed was for her to say, 'You can quit.' If she agreed, my guilt would be minimum. If she didn't agree, I'd be guilt-ridden the rest of my life. Convoluted? Yes. But I was miserable and still crying. She smiled that therapist smile that translates to 'knock it off,' "Look, they need you and you are learning from them."

"What am I learning?" I squeaked out. "How to fall apart? How to get dehydrated? How to live inside death?" I didn't say any of that. Nietzsche kept running through my mind, "Out of life's school of war – what doesn't kill me, makes me stronger."[27] Oh-yeah-sure-right.

Forty-five minutes later, "Keep leading the group, it won't kill you, you'll learn."

I left her office. Maybe I need a new supervisor. "What will I learn?" I announced into the air sounding younger than four on 91st Street. After pouting for a block or so, I forced myself to return to adulthood. I knew quitting would set a sorry precedent. Would I quit my patients when things got difficult? Would I quit learning psychoanalysis? Would I start quitting whenever something upset me? Would I stop/quit trusting in myself?

Do you remember that feeling when you were about to ride a rollercoaster for the first time? You wait and wait for people to get out of the way because you're a kid and need to be first. You want the front seat because it's first and because you have no idea what's going to happen. As the rollercoaster clanks up that first hill, that large really big hill that provides impetus for the rest of the ride, you realize when you're at the very tippy top of the hill, now you see what you've done to yourself. The incredible headfirst straight downhill ride, that if you live, you'll be stronger and wiser. The moral of this story: "Let her run the group by herself. She'll learn humility." That GMHC administrator gave me the front seat on the rollercoaster.

Now, walking away from my supervisor's office, I felt traumatized by her decree and the ice-cold windy weather wasn't helping. New York has monstrous winds in late winter, and I wasn't in the mood to walk to my office. I decided to hail a taxi. Whenever there's weather in New York City and whenever you need to get somewhere fast, there are no taxis. There are no taxis available during the daytime or when it's dark, or during a weekday or on a weekend. If it's raining, or snowing, or too hot, or too cold, or even 'just right,' taxi drivers don't feel like driving because there are too many customers.

Unable to wave down a taxi, I had to walk twenty minutes to my office. After the first few blocks, I came to the cross streets of 86th and Columbus Avenue. This is a notorious wind tunnel street that stretches from the East River to the Hudson River. While waiting for the cross-the-street 'walk' light to appear, I moseyed toward the corner newspaper stand, and leaned over to read the headlines. In this exact lean-over-glance-at-headline moment, a powerful gust of wind whipped around the 86th Street and Columbus Avenue and reached its pinacol in front of the newsstand. This maelstrom wind is the kind that totally flips people's hair, so your bangs no longer cover any part of your forehead. Then, as you're repositioning your bangs you realize your blue very large swing coat is about to attack your briefcase. (This is the message in the song *Tangled Up in Blue*. *Blowin' in the Wind* would work here, too. As would *Idiot Wind*. Thank you, Bob Dylan) All this and more happened the very same concurrent exact moment.

Perhaps it was due to the alignment of the planets or my morning pills or my supervisor's stubbornness, that I was totally exhausted by 8:45 AM. As such, I was no match for this Banshee Columbus and 86th Street windstorm. It swished my blue swing coat *and* my briefcase between my legs.

An aside: 86th Street and Columbus Avenue are very close to the subway stop where mobs of people exit in morning rush hour, which happens to be right now, so quite a few of those subway exiting people are all headed toward the corner newsstand which is next to the war between my clothing, accessories, and newspaper headlines.

Splat! Down I go! Right in the middle of everything. In hindsight, I wished I'd fallen gently, in that Pavlova dying swan position. Instead, it was a splat! First my butt met the sidewalk, then my back. There I was, staring up at the blue sky until an older woman leaned over me, "Do you need help?"

"No, I'm fine." Seriously, are you going to let an old woman, on a crowded street corner pick you up, probably drop you, then join you on the ground? I braced myself between the sidewalk and the wind and slowly took the downward facing dog yoga pose followed by the salute to the sun yoga pose. When I was upright, I wondered if the reason I fell was payback. If I had spent the money and not sneakily tried to get a free glance at the newspaper headlines, I wouldn't have fallen. Karma.

Once again on both feet, I knew something was wrong. My first step didn't work. I decided my legs were probably in shock after the briefcase/blue swing coat battle and my feet were just confused. I was too humiliated to ask for help and forced myself to move. My left foot made a crunch sound. As a psychoanalyst, I decided the pain was in my head and forced myself to walk to my office. The twenty-minute walk to my office took forty-five. Limping takes a little longer.

Chapter 32
Getting Plastered

The first patient of the day arrived moments after I limped into my office. During the session, I noted my foot was ballooning. Fifteen minutes later, my foot had morphed over the sides of my shoe. My patient didn't notice the now mammoth ball at the end of my leg. Half an hour later, she left. I hopped to my desk, called and canceled my other patients of the day, grabbed my hostile blue swing coat, hopped 'up' the stairs to the street and by a stroke of luck or maybe it was the pill alignment, hailed a taxi.

"Where to, lady?"

"Lenox Hill Hospital, the Emergency Room." I had a good relationship with this hospital. They were very kind when I arrived after a bicycle ran into me last year.

To get from the Westside of Manhattan to the Eastside during the shank end of the rush hour in a matter of minutes is amazing. I hopped out of the taxi, then hopped into the hospital's Emergency Room. Whomever was in charge immediately sent a wheelchair accompanied by a nurse. The staff was really nice, very attentive, and very efficient. This became clear when I realized my level of insurance was Cadillac.

In no time at all, I'm on the X-ray bed.

"Well, if you look right here on the X-ray, you'll see this line. Your fifth metatarsal bone is broken."

"Noooooo."

"Yessssss."

"How did that happen? Did someone step on your foot?"

"Yes. My right foot stepped on the outside part of my left foot."

"Well, that's interesting. Your right foot reached over and stepped on the far side of your left foot. That makes for a very interesting visual, I think." The doctor smiled and told me to wait, he'd be right back. Where did he think my good foot would hop me to? Why would I leave a hospital with a ridiculously mutilated fifth metatarsal?

A couple minutes later, another doctor arrived. He was armed by two medical gurney-pushers. They pushed me into a small but nicely furnished three-sided room. The fourth side was a dainty Liberty-print privacy curtain which they closed so no one could see me. As a result, I had no idea what was coming next. To my surprise, it was another doctor accompanied by a bucket full of plaster. He sat down very close to my foot and I could tell he wanted to touch it. I'm afraid to look at it much less touch it.

"What are you doing?"

"We need to plaster your foot."

"Why."

"It's broken."

"I know that."

"We have to plaster it. It needs to be immobilized so you don't further injure it."

"Oh, don't worry. I won't further injure it. Thank you. I don't want a plaster cast." He smiled and left the room. Five minutes later he returned with a whole team of doctors, all of them smiling and staring at me as they created a horizontal line-up in front of me. What happened to the Liberty-print privacy curtain? Realistically, at this point there was no need for the privacy curtain. The row of onlooking doctors provided a wall of white coats.

"What's going on?"

"We're going to put your foot in a plaster cast."

"You need an army of white jackets to do that?" White jackets in my profession get a bad (w)rap, no pun intended.

"Why do you need such a big bucket of plaster?" I was exasperated, "Doctor, I don't want a plaster cast as I've previously mentioned to you. Doctor, you are missing the point of why I'm here. Keep your plaster and you can keep my broken foot, too. Just give me a new foot and I'm good to go."

The white wall was closing in on me. I assume they were interested in this continuing education course of 'how to make plaster.' The doctor took advantage of my distraction and sneakily started plastering my foot. Then, miraculously all the white coats parted, like that Moses parted the Red Sea moment. There he is, another white coat bringing a pair of wooden crutches.

"Are you kidding? I don't know how to drive those things and you know very well that I can barely walk on two good feet or I wouldn't be here now."

My frustration was mounting, "Doctor, do you really think I can walk plastered, with a broken foot, and this wooden impingement? Do you know how windy it is out there? What happens if there's more weather and I'm out there wearing plaster and wood?"

"We'll teach you how to use the crutches after we finish getting you plastered."

In the early 1990s, plaster on a broken foot meant you've got stark-white plaster smooshed onto the broken body part. It's smooshed from your toes right up to your knee, which is seriously overdoing it.

The doctor was good for his word. He taught me how to drive the crutch before saying goodbye. I left the hospital, crutched to the corner and hailed a taxi. My luck was amazing. Two successfully hailed taxis in one day. Totally, unheard of in Manhattan. I couldn't wait to tell my friends.

"Where to, miss?"

"I want to go home. Upper westside, 88th Street, off the park."

"What happened to you? Did you get hit by a bicycle?"

"No, that was last time, a year ago." Then curiously, "Why? Were you my taxi driver when the bike ran over me?"

"No. I don't keep a record of passengers."

"The reason I went to Lenox Hill hospital was that I stepped on myself. My right foot stepped onto my left foot in a sort of miraculously juxtaposed manner."

"Wow!"

"It's quite a visual, I know."

I arrived at my apartment. Apartments in New York City are well aware elevators rarely work and I live on the sixth floor. I decided to use my enormous blue swing coat, as a reverse sliding board and scrooch up each stairwell stair, one butt-step at a time. Finally, I arrive at my apartment and realize it is not broken-foot-proofed. High gloss polyurethane floors, sunken living room, coffee table directly in front of the couch you want to lie on.

Then it hit me. This foot catastrophe is a legitimate excuse to quit GMHC. Never mind, that won't work. Everyone in the group has a physical handicap and they come to group no matter how crappy they feel. I'll just limp it out.

I had some experience limping during childhood. During recuperation from my tonsillectomy, I realized I had to refill the ice cream bowl. Enroute I heard my parents stifling laughter. "Why are you limping?"

I was shocked. "I just had my tonsils out!" My parents forgot? They drove me to the hospital, for goodness sake.

"Tonsillectomies don't make people limp," Dad said chuckling.

I struck back, "Dad, everyone limps after an operation."

"Okay, Chester," he retorted.

I continued limping and whining a little bit until I reached the Hotpoint refrigerator. "Dad, Chester limped after he had an operation. Dad, we watched that episode of *Gun Smoke*, together." Pause. "Dad, you know Chester limped on *Gun Smoke*."

"Dennis Weaver didn't really limp."

Unbelievable! Dad was demented at twenty-eight years old.

"Dad, *Gun Smoke,* Marshal Matt Dillon, 10:00 Tuesday nights." I refueled the ice cream bowl from the five by ten-inch ice box and ditched the return limp to not further embarrass my dad. Amazing, even though Dad watched

Gun Smoke he didn't know it created preexisting conditions.

Chapter 33
Shoeless

Wednesday, late March 1990. My crutch hailed a taxi and we headed to GMHC. This was the evening Da-veed and Raul were joining the group. I wanted to arrive early to not draw attention to my plaster and crutch. But, as each person entered, my plastered foot/leg received glowing accolades.

"What happened?" Jason's smile became concerned.

"I broke my foot. I'm fine. I have to keep it elevated."

"Here," he grabbed a chair for foot elevation.

"What happened to you?" Neil looked worried.

"Stepped on myself."

"What?" Jason muttered, looping his arm around the back of my chair. "What happened?" I'd never heard Jason speak with such gentleness.

"Well, I danced a tango with Mariah, I mean with the wind last week."

"Tangled?"

"No. It was more isomorphic than that. I stepped on myself." Jason smiled compassionately.

"You see," I descriptively continued. "My right foot thought it was my left foot." He nodded, so I went on.

"You're right, Jason. It wasn't tango. It was more like a Riverdance soloist at the Edinburg Fringe Festival." I can't believe I said that. Riverdance is *not* Scottish, for god's sake. I didn't say. Back to the point: "My right foot stepped on my left foot and right after that, I got plastered at Lenox Hill Hospital." Jason chucked; his arm remained around my chair. Then, he motioned to Neil to get my crutch which meant it made the rounds, as baton, fencing sword, pogo stick, and various other playthings. Perhaps Jason's demeanor changed in relation to my physical vulnerability. It didn't rival his, of course, but pain needs companions.

As things settled down, i.e., when they finally put my crutch in the corner, I was about to begin.

"Where's Chris?" Neil asked.

"Here! I'm here." Chris flew into the room, out of breath, panting, "I ran to get here." He sat down, still breathing heavily.

I began again, "We have two new members today. Let's start off this evening with introduuu…"

Chris interrupted while still trying to catch his breath, "Sorry. I just got a phone call from Fernando's caretaker." In the next second, the cadence of Chris' voice stalled, then cracked, then wheezed.

"Fernando died last Thursday. His caretaker called me this afternoon. Did she call you?"

"I've been in meetings today. I haven't checked my messages," I mumbled.

Chris' eyes were swollen and red. Perhaps from the cold wind or crying. Probably both.

"Wait! He died the day *after* he was here?" Neil looked horrified.

Chris struggled to speak, "I'm sorry." He was looking at the two new members. "I'm sorry you new people have to hear this in your first session." Chris' voice stumbled again, "Fernando loved this group. His caretaker said he talked more about us than his family."

Jason interjected, "He had a special place in this group. You guys agree, right?" They nodded. The mood sank into silence.

After a few moments, I asked the group, "Would anyone like to say more about Fernando? About what you're feeling?" No one responded.

Neil took over, "If we talk about his death, it will make it more real."

Jason quickly reacted, then clearing his throat, "Speaking for myself, this isn't new. We're always losing someone we care about. It's what we know. I mean this happens all the time to us." He sighed, "Death is different now. It's different than before the virus. It's just a matter of time." I don't think Jason's head could have hung any lower. He looked miserable. We all did.

Then, composing himself, "I don't know. I don't want to speak for the group. Do any of you want to talk about Fernando?" Jason murmured.

They all looked defeated, except the new members. They were just absorbing, probably.

"I think we'll always talk about Fernando or hold him in our mind, our hearts." My voice sounded toneless, lost. I kept trying, "Perhaps this loss is more intense, as it's additionally fueled from losing Thomas and Matthew."

"Could we talk about this some other time?" Jason sighed. The group silently agreed.

I concurred. "We have two new people here. Let's begin with introductions."

Neil glanced at the two new members, "Okay, you guys tell us about yourselves." Raul looked apprehensive; Da-veed didn't.

To equalize intent, I added, "You know you'll all have to introduce yourselves, but for this evening, let's hear from our two new members."

I smiled, then asked, "Da-veed, Raul, who wants to go first?"

Chapter 34
The House of Da-veed

It began with Da-veed waving his hand the way the British Royals do, in conjunction with a long haughty scoot to the edge of his folding chair. Then in a voice loud enough for the audience to hear at the back of the theater even if you're sitting way up in the balcony nose-bleed section, he announced, "I'll go first." His words felt abrasive, sort of like a rabbit punch, or more specifically like an unwanted penetration. Clearly, he was oblivious to the group's mood as well as his too-quick reaction about 'going first.' At that moment, I found myself mentally flipping pages in the DSM (*Diagnostic Statistic Manual*) because who is this guy? He seemed so different than when I interviewed him. Where was he hiding this part of him?

Struggling to find empathy, not sure if it was for him or me, I decided to rationalize, 'He's new.' Then I came up with a pretty good analytic interpretation, i.e., perhaps his obliviousness is unconscious, a defense against feeling fearful or anxious. Some people deal with anxiety through dissociation. They tune out, emotionally shut down sounds and surroundings. That could be it. No, it wasn't. It was just plain old narcissism. In the next second, Da-veed slid his body to the back on his chair and cheerfully announced, "Are y'all ready for me?"

"Yeah," Jason acrimoniously responded. "We're ready and waiting."

Neil folded his arms over his chest and announced, "This is going to be precious." Neil's sarcasm rolled right off Da-veed's back as he dismissively snapped his fingers and winked at Neil.

"Oh, I am just so used to jealousy, honey."

"*Whoa!*" I thought. What? Was Da-veed pretending or faking sensitivity when I interviewed him? He was certainly performing insensitivity now. Either way, I felt duped. In addition, his mannerisms had become flamboyantly feminine. This too, was not evident during the interview.

Da-veed's presentation (of self) was overly dramatic, or histrionic at the least. For instance, he didn't cross his legs, he crossed his ankles in a very delicate manner, exactly the way I learned in Charm School. His face was mesmerizing because he championed that suck-in-your-cheeks-look-to-show-off-the-sunken-cheek-bone-look. His skin was incredibly milky, chocolate milky. He had huge eyes bookended by false eyelashes that fluttered for emphasis. His brown wavy hair fell to his shoulders, allowing frequent flips between fingers. Da-veed's body was willowy and somehow swayed in time with the cadence of his voice. He was quite beautiful and more feminine than I am, which is no easy feat.

"Da-veed, you don't need to raise your hand to speak, we just try not to talk over each other," I was referencing his British Royal hand-wave. He smiled, then literally sang out, "Oh, thank you. I'll do just that." Chris had the most visibly negative expression than anyone else in the room, which is saying something. Maybe Chris was wondering if the room was big enough for two singers. Da-veed inhaled to swell his voice, probably the way Jimmy Stewart did in the movie *Mr. Smith Goes to Washington*, except it won't go well if Da-veed starts to filibuster.

"This is an AIDS group," Da-veed announced, grinning. Everyone had that 'duh' expression. "I was diagnosed with full-blown AIDS in 1986 after my PCP bout of pneumonia. Y'all know what I mean, right?" A few group members revisited the 'duh' expression, others seemed mesmerized with Da-veed's hair swishing. It had that Rita Hayworth *Gilda* quality.

Da-veed shook his long curls then tucked some behind one ear, sat up straight-er, swung his torso left to right until assured he had everyone's attention.

Smiling, inauthentically, "You want to know a little about me?" Not waiting for an answer, "Of course you do. Do any of you recognize me?"

Gilda? I didn't say that out loud.

Da-veed's face beamed, "Darlings, I am sure you've been to a ball, right?"

It was already apparent Da-veed's questions were rhetorical. "You know about Pepper LaBeija, Paris Dupree, Octavia St. Laurent, right? Well, honey, I have 'walked' with these gorgeous queens at our balls."

Neil somehow interrupted, "I've been there, not to 'walk,' just watch."

"Honey, then you got an eye full!"

With mounting affect Da-veed lavishly continued, "Oh! The fashions! The awards for beauty! The fantastic talented individuals! Everyone is a star! A diva! Beautiful! Gorgeous!" Da-veed punctuated each exclamation mark with a French fingertip kiss that ended with, "Magnifique!"

"Maybe he's a Francophile," I thought, hoping he wouldn't want to double kiss cheeks at the end of the session.

"The ball is everything. A world in itself. A place for people to be whoever they want." He took a deep breath, "What I love about the balls are the competitions. Oh, the voguing is fantastic. But you have to perform. You have to pass as real. It's all about 'realness.' You know what I mean, y'all?" Another rhetorical question. "Let me tell you what I'm talking about." Da-veed was looking directly at me, obviously thinking I didn't know what he was talking about, which was totally true. "There's one competitive category called Business Executive. If you're competing in this category, you have to pass. I mean, if you walked out on the street (which isn't done), people on the street have to believe you *are* a business executive. It's the same thing for each category. The best category, according to me, is runway modeling. Voguing on the runway. The clothes! A lot of people sew their own gowns for this competition and they're breathtaking." Da-veed sat back without intent to relinquish the floor.

What'd I tell you? Here comes Jimmy Stewart's filibustering.

"During a ball, you achieve your highest level of perfection. You are who you choose to be. Except, honey, you have to be queer and 'of color.' A ball is where nobody's rejected for being who or what they want to be. Those of us who walk, well, we belong to the ball." He scanned the group checking our attention. "Oh, there's more, honey. Let me tell you." Da-veed gushed, "Oh, my, my, my! These balls would make y'all feel like it's *you* who don't belong." With that, Da-veed pointed at everyone individually, his finger rhythmically moving like the bouncing ball in sing-along cartoons. No one in the group was smiling let alone singing. "No lily-white boys are allowed to 'walk.' Y'all can come watch us, but it's only Latinos and Blacks who can walk. We reign. The balls are about us and for us."

Neil interrupted, "You've won trophies, I take it?" Da-veed swelled with pride which didn't seem possible due to his ongoing mounting hubris.

"Of course! I've received many trophies, honey. A great big trophy for passing in the beauty category. Oh, girl, that is one of the most difficult trophies to get. I wore a pastel periwinkle unbelievably sequined gown." At that moment, Da-veed nodded in my direction probably checking if I envied his gown.

"Don't worry, I'm good with the gowns I have."

Da-veed gently stroked his face, ignored my comment, and continued his monologue, "I went to Paris' Ball in 1986. *I* was in the audience when Paris Dupree announced, 'Butch queen!' I mean, it was *her* ball. She could say whatever she wanted. So, Paris yells out, she yells, 'Boy by day, girl by night.'" Da-veed stopped and put both hands over his heart as though he was going to faint from admiration or whatever. Then, he belted out a loud, 'ohhhhhhh!' which reminded me of the 1953 movie where Jeanette MacDonald and Nelson Eddy loudly sang into each other's face in *Indian Love Call*.

Da-veed's attention landed on me again, "Do you know what I'm talking about?"

"Ahhh, maybe?"

With bubbling condescension, "Oh, no you don't, dear. I'll explain some other time, honey."

My backbone bolted up quicker than a stock market rise on a Friday evening right before a three day weekend. "Actually, Da-veed, I use my first name, not 'dear' or 'honey.'" Da-veed was either oblivious to professional boundaries or didn't give a hoot. "Oh, poo! I forgot myself," he said slightly smirking. "Well, let's face it, my dear, I know you don't know any of this, so I'm explaining as best I can."

Da-veed was gaining grandiosity lickety split. "Only someone who *actually* goes to the balls and 'walks' knows what I'm talking about." Da-veed haughtily continued, "Getting back to Paris. Well, Paris Dupree created a category for wannabe drag queens, first timers who walk at a ball. Very generous of her, you know."

Suddenly, Da-veed clapped his hands and nearly flew off his chair with excitement. "I bet none of you know *thi*s! I know none of you know about the movie."

With superiority swelling like a tsunami, which seemed impossible to improve on, Da-veed excitedly announced, "Let me tell you all about the movie. None of you know about the movie they're making about drag." Another rhetorical question. "You'll never believe this. There's a movie being filmed about us, about the balls. They're interviewing some of the mothers."

Neil added, "I know the documentary you're talking about. They've been filming it for a while now."

"Well, honey, they have already filmed some of the balls and you'll see what I'm talking about. The clothes the mothers' wear are gorgeous. My favorite is Octavia St. Laurent. Oh, sweetie, she is just the best mother as far as I'm concerned, the absolute best. When she 'walks' she's queen of queens."

"Wait. What you mean by mothers," I interrupted.

Da-veed grinned, "Well, honey, oops. I called you honey again. I can't call you honey?"

"That's right, you can't call her honey," Jason angrily interjected.

Da-veed didn't blink or miss a beat. "Mothers are angels of the street. They take the young gay boys who are living on the street into their house *if* they have potential to 'walk.' They train the boys how to pass at the balls and win trophies. After you win a lot of trophies and make some money, you can start your own house, but that's a lot of work. Well, thank heaven, we have established mothers because they will take you under their wing. Mothers can take the young hustlers off the street if they think they'll do well at a ball. They feed them, give them a roof over their head, they give the boys a family. There are a lot of reasons why a mother could take you in, but usually it's because they think you have what it takes to 'walk.' Mothers provide a place to get trained. Now let me explain what a house is." Once again, he looked at me and why was he repeating himself? "Every house has a mother and maybe a father and siblings. No one's related, though, and everyone is queer."

Jason interjected, "Da-veed, do you need some air? You're working up a sweat?"

Perhaps in leu of getting more air, Da-veed waved his hand as though holding *Lady Windermere's Fan.* Oscar Wilde would have been outrageously pleased.

"No, no, I'm coooool! I am cool! So, coooool. I just might be in the movie."

"It's a documentary," Neil corrected.

Da-veed swung around and flirtatiously asked, "What's your name, honey?"

Neil folded his arms over his chest and leaned back. Then, without emotionality, Neil responded, "Neil."

Everyone in the group appeared so outrageously angry their folding chairs began to rattle. I decided to interrupt, in hopes of containing a hostile takeover aimed at Da-veed. It felt like the group, unconsciously and collectively, were enacting reaction formation: Anger toward Da-veed replaced sorrow about Fernando.

"Thank you for the introduction, D-veed. Your background sounds quite glamorous. A fantasy world that creates realness in 'passing.' It's especially interesting and wonderful that the mothers provide a type of personalized social service."

"Oh, they do! They help so many boys. Those poor boys. That's why I said the mothers are angels."

"Thank you, Da-veed. We don't have too much time left, so let's hear from Raul," I introjected.

"Oh, no, there's more. Mucho more." Seriously? Da-veed sideswiped me? Unfortunately, I had to sideswipe back, otherwise he'd kidnap the session again.

"I understand there's more, but we need to hear from Raul."

Unfazed, Da-veed continued, "I just want to finish what I'm talking about. I haven't finished."

"We need to leave time for Raul."

Once again, environmentally immune, Da-veed kept talking. "The pièce de resistance..." Da-veed dramatically inhaled, probably an attempt to create a pregnant cliffhanger moment.

Jason leaned into my left ear and whispered, "I don't like him. He won't fit."

"Hummmm," was the best I could muster. Who the is this guy? Did I interview his twin and not this grandiose kidnapper person?

"So!" Da-veed's voice became louder. "Here's the pièce de résistance!"

"Another one?" Jason sarcastically sneered.

Da-veed kept right on trucking. "Like I said before I was rudely interrupted, this movie is being filmed during some of the balls and a few mothers are going to be interviewed."

"*David*, she said we've only got a few more minutes and we still have to hear from Raul." Jason's voice was loud and stern.

"The name, darling is Da-veed, not David." Da-veed dismissively continued, "Anyway, the movie, I mean the documentary as you all are intent on calling it, is supposed to be released in 1991."

Jason's body stiffened, "David, before you 'walked,' you were in one of these houses, right? You said that mothers take in gay boys who are on the street, hustling."

"That's right."

"Did you hustle before getting into a house?"

"Of course, darling."

"You don't turn tricks anymore, do you? You don't hustle anymore, right?"

Da-veed stared at Jason, then angrily scoffed, "What do you think I do, sweetie."

Jason stared back, "I'm serious. Do you still hustle?"

With flippant hostility, "A girl has to feed herself."

"Not by hustling. Do you still hustle?" Jason aggressively challenged.

"You stopped hustling when you got AIDS, right?" Neil was joining Jason's fury.

Silence.

Jason took back the mantel, "Are you still on the 'street?'"

Da-veed's silence was steaming hot. He stared at Jason as though boring a hole through him.

Chris broke in, "Da-veed, we're just asking if you continued hustling after diagnosis."

"I know what ya'll are asking. Did I ask you who you infected? How many boys did you infect? Huh? Are you telling me you got infected and, opps, just stopped messing around? Oh, but the difference is you poor creatures weren't asking for money, right?" Dripping with indignant sarcasm and mockery, "Like I'm hustling and making people pay to get AIDS, isn't that right, sweeties? Yeah, that's what I'm doing. That's right."

Da-veed's arrogant aggression felt overwhelming. Suddenly, he pointed at Jason and Neil and hostilely taunted, "You two are incredibly naive. What kind of job do you think I could get? A job at a bank, or a restaurant?"

With scoffing superiority, "Don't get your bloomers all twisted up."

Jason's fury peaked, "What the hell? So, you are? You *are* hustling when you know you've got AIDS?"

"Getting paid the big bucks, honey." Da-veed's sarcasm thickened with ridicule. "If I could get a job, a real job, don't you think I would? Get paid regular. You gonna hire me? Come on. Would you hire me? Honey, I didn't even go to high school. Who's going to hire a gay black kid from the ghetto who didn't finish school? I was on the street at thirteen. Let me tell you, as bad as the street is, it's better than living with my aunt and whatever passing-by-flavor-of-the-month boyfriend she's got and her four kids."

Suddenly, Da-veed seemed to change tact, going full force for sympathy. "She's got a steady stream of druggies, pushers, pimps. Nobody cared when I left home, if that's what you want to call it. I left, lived on the street until I heard about the balls. Until I got taught how to 'walk.' We had food on the table at mother's house, nobody was using, and nobody was going to beat the crap out of you."

Jason reacted angrily, "I get it. It was tough for you to grow up. That's not the point, are you still turning tricks knowing you're *positive*?"

"Yeah, are you *still* hustling?" Neil's voice pitched.

"Da-veed, just tell us if you're still hustling. We just want to know if you're still turning tricks," Chris' voice cracked.

In a mocking sing-song tone, Da-veed angrily snapped back, "Honey, I make a lot of money doing what I do."

Neil's face and neck were flushed from anger. Jason was ready to spit nails. Chris looked worn out, his chin inches from his chest. Everyone looked disgusted, especially Da-veed.

"Enough! Stop," I loudly interjected. "This has been a way too bumpy night. Disagree with each other, but let's stop slinging insults."

Da-veed looked around, took a deep breath and with fury and contempt, let it rip, "Okay, girls. Y'all so full of yourselves, so damn full of yourselves. No, I don't hustle anymore. If I was white, would you automatically question that? Y'all just made up your minds that I must be some piece of shit, going around infecting people."

Da-veed scornfully smirked, "Y'all just decided that. You made up your mind and decided you were right. I'm some slut sharing my AIDS."

"Stop. Everyone stop," my voice was loud and angry.

Da-veed ignored me and continued taunting, "Do you girls think Da-veed is going to leave here tonight and go directly to the piers?" He smacked his knee. "That's what you think? Am I right? That's what you think, and you don't even know me. Y'all disgust me."

Jason almost shot up from his chair.

"Jason, I'll manage it. I'll manage it," I repeated emphatically.

"Honey, I'm fine. Don't worry about me." Then, Da-veed once again pointed at Neil and Jason. "It's you two, you two high and all-mighty, both of you. You're so critical of someone you don't even know."

Da-veed's anger slid him to the edge of his chair. He stared at Jason, then at Neil, "I'm not going to sit through this sorry group." Da-veed grabbed his coat. "Y'all disgust me. You hear me? I'm disgusted." Da-veed stomped to the doorway, then turned around for a final shot, "I feel sorry for y'all. Y'all have to tolerate these two." He dramatically swung around and stormed out, leaving the hallway to echo indigent furry.

Chapter 35
Raul

"Would you like to discuss what happened or move on?"

Unanimous, "Move on."

"Raul, how you doing? Are you alright?" I asked.

"Yeah, just listening. Just listening."

"That interaction didn't make you rethink joining the group?"

"No, none of that was directed at me. I'm fine." Raul reacted as though nothing happened. "My name is Raul and I was diagnosed with AIDS in 1986. I am not on AZT and whatnot."

"Raul, what do you mean by whatnot?" Jason abruptly interjected.

"You know, research on AZT isn't solid. A lot of people don't know much about it, and I don't want to be a guinea pig before I know it's safe. Some people are saying that taking AZT gets worse, you know? I mean, this is just me. Just how I think and that's it."

Neil cut in, "Most of us are on a low dose of AZT."

Raul seemed unfazed, "A lot of people on the west coast are not taking it. You can do whatever you want, but there are lots of skeptics on what AZT does. This is just my opinion. I think it's dangerous to take it when we don't know much about how it works."

"True. We don't know how it works. I don't know how my antidepressant works, either." Neil reacted with a tinge of mockery.

Raul shot back, "Oh, come on. Didn't you guys read the articles on AZT in *The New York Native*?[27] They've published a bunch of articles on AZT, and they say it's poison."[28]

"I had no idea the staff at the *Native* have medical degrees," Jason quipped.

"No, look you guys, they've likened using it to what Nazi Germany did to *undesirables* and whatnot. Gays are undesirable."

Chris tried to lighten the mood, "I've met a lot of gay men who are totally desirable."

"Good try, Chris," Neil interjected.

In contrast and indifference, Raul continued, "There's so much focus on AZT that no one is looking for other medications. Do you really believe that there's no antiviral med that's been on the market before now?" Raul scoffed, "All of a sudden there's a cancerous virus and, oops, we don't have any med for this.' There's no hard data on what AZT does. You all know that. I think it's toxic and just makes things worse, and whatnot."

Jason caustically mumbled, "I'm still confused about 'whatnot.'"

Raul looked around, "You guys are caught up with what's the best AZT milligram to take, you're not looking at its toxicity."

"Who said we aren't looking at toxicity?" Jason harshly challenged.

"Weren't you saying someone just died? What was his name? Fernando, right? Was he taking AZT?" Raul looked incredulous, "You know AZT played a part in that, right? Look, AZT is a cancer drug. It's supposed to kill cancer cells, and whatnot. That's what it does. Some doctors say it kills white blood cells. They think that's why people taking AZT become anemic. I read that AZT depletes red blood cells. It attacks white blood cells *and* red blood cells."

At this point, I was exhausted, and the others looked in a similar funk. "Guys, we've gone over our session time. I'm sorry to cut you off, Raul, but we need to end the session."

"Yeah, let's end this ridiculous discussion," Neil abruptly broke in.

"A ridiculous discussion thanks to you and Da-veed," Jason jabbed.

Raul's skin flushed deep red from unleased anger as he stood up, aggressively swung his coat barely missing Chris' head, and stormed out the door.

"You guys done?" The janitor asked Raul as they passed in the hallway.

Raul angrily shouted down the hallway, "Oh, they are unbelievably done. *They're* history."

Chapter 36
Listening to the Unspoken

It was April 1990 and as usual, I went home to Pennsylvania for the Easter holiday, but this time Easter was overshadowed by my mother's terminal breast cancer. She was now bedridden, fed through a tube, on a morphine drip, and breathing only with the help of oxygen. It was a too-loud oxygen machine that kept my father awake at night and as a result, my mother and the loud oxygen machine removed themselves to my childhood bedroom.

I remember the dread I felt that Easter day as I climbed the stairs to my old bedroom. I peeked in. There she was, a once beautiful, tall woman with blonde hair and green eyes, now diminished, destroyed by cancer, chemo, and radiation. Only her green eyes remained loyal. Her shrunken body was lying on the spare twin bed in my old room. She was transfixed by the television. "What's the movie, Mom?"

"Shirley Temple, *The Little Princess*." This was Shirley Temple's first technicolor film that my mother was watching on a black and white TV in my room.

"I'll watch it with you," I said hobbling to the other twin bed. My broken foot, plaster cast and me were her constant companions that day. We were frequently double-checked by everyone home for the holiday. Mid-day my mother passed away in a room full of tears from family and friends.

Three weeks after her burial, I returned to New York. It was now spring, 1990. Somehow, the months of April and May mysteriously hide February and March weather within them, creating opportunity for mourning to sink further into any abyss.

A few days later, I went to GMHC. Long Eyelashes no longer graced the reception desk. With plaster and wood, I crutched to the elevator, crutched a little more through the hallway and entered my group room.

Throughout the life of the group, I sat next to Jason. On this evening, he seemed smaller and less agile than three weeks ago. He smiled as I took my seat, then in a gentle tone, "Your mother died."

I was shocked, "How do you know? How do you know it was my mother?"

"Experience."

I was speechless.

Again, Jason heard the unspoken. "I know mourning when I see it." My stomach sank into vulnerability.

"We only have three people tonight," Jason's voice was weak and husky.

I glanced at Neil. His skin was much grayer then when I last saw him.

"I'm sorry you lost your mother." Neil tried to smile, but it seemed painful.

"How are you doing, Chris?" I gently solicited. Chris still 'looked' untouched by AZT or AIDS.

"I'm good. Sorry about your mother."

"It's good to be back and I'm very glad to see the three of you. Oh, you probably already know this, when I called GMHC to tell them I would be absent due to a family emergency, the administrator told me Da-veed and Raul were not coming back to our group."

"Oh, thank the lord," Neil sighed.

His rejoicing was seconded by Jason and Chris.

"It's just us now," I whispered. Tentatively, "Should I interview more men?"

"No." A triplet unanimous response.

Neil exhaled, "It's too hard and it's too late. The three of us agreed, no more new people. We talked about it before you got here tonight. No more new people."

Two years ago, there were three empty chairs at our first session. Now, there are only three chairs occupied. Why was it always three?

Jason leaned closer, "We made another decision. This is our last meeting. We want to dissolve our group."

"Alright," I slowly responded, apprehensively.

"We also decided you won't create another group."

"I won't or I shouldn't?"

"Both."

"You mean because my mother died?"

"That wasn't the reason we made the decision. We decided you're done."

"Isn't that my decision?"

"No," Jason mumbled.

"We know this has become too hard for you to manage," Chris' voice was tender.

"How did you know? Well, of course you know." My face was flushed, and I was struggling to keep my voice steady. "How long have my emotions been cellophane?"

"We could feel it. We know you," Jason mumbled.

I couldn't look at their faces, if I did, I'd cry. Oh, I can't believe it! Why am I trying to not cry? I felt my shoulders drop. Hadn't I learned anything from these men? I forced myself to look at them and said, "I'm going to cry."

Chris reacted first, "So are we."

Jason picked up the box of tissues to give me, but first stalled to take some for himself. Then he passed the tissue box to Chris, then to Neil and finally to me. For a few moments, we four used way too many tissues.

Neil chuckled, "I didn't think we'd do this. That we'd all cry. I knew *I* would, though."

I looked at my remaining three and sadly confessed, "I hear what the three of you have said. I will not run another group."

"Good," Neil said emphatically. Chris and Jason nodded approval.

Moving to the edge of my chair, I sighed to the point I felt no air in my lungs. "There is something I'd like to talk about. Since we met, the group has been protecting me. In one of our first group sessions, you insisted I not to visit when you get hospitalized. You said if I went, I'd burn out. So, I never said goodbye to anyone in the group, except Fernando, I guess." Then it hit me. They were right. It was seeing Fernando last days that began my burn out. They were absolutely right and so I told them, they were right.

"If you said goodbye to everyone, you wouldn't have made it."

"We barely knew each other back then. How'd you know?"

Jason chuckled, "I knew what it was like to run this kind of group."

Feeling incredibly vulnerable, "Right. You knew, but I sure didn't. I didn't know what I was doing back then."

Jason responded, "Yeah, that was obvious."

"It was?"

"No, I'm kidding. Most of us didn't know how to be in a group, either."

"Did I look like I needed protection?"

Neil smiled, "Early on, I think we all white knuckled it."

Chris added, "I remember your face when Vito showed us his address book. You were very emotional. Your face was flushed."

"You mean like it is right now?"

Jason smiled, "Just like now, yes."

"There was another powerful session. It was almost overwhelming," I recounted.

"Which one?" Chris asked.

"I'm not sure what the topic was. I couldn't look at anyone, so I stared at the flowers on my dress. Somehow, I took an emotional vacation during that session. I kept thinking about a park in Norway. It was full of roses. Just like the dress I was wearing. During the session, my mind drifted back to a beautiful garden. Actually, the garden isn't the important part. There was a path through the garden that led to an obelisk. It was a huge granite obelisk made up of life-size naked bodies; grown men. I think the bodies were male. They were curled up, like a fetus, one fetus body resting on top of the next. There were more than a hundred male bodies piled forty-five feet into the sky. The obelisk reminded me of how you have supported each other, leaned on one another and how tenderly eight men melted into a group. This obelisk of male bodies, the heaviness of each body must be similar to the emotional weight you carried each day, for and with each other."

How in the world did my eight men emotionally manage to support each other? Weren't they burdened by the succession of deaths? Weren't they overwhelmed waiting for their own demise.

I heard myself say, "Let's never end this session."

"I agree," Chris responded.

"I need to go home and I don't want to, but I need to," Jason lamented. "Chris, would you get my coat. My leg is really hurting. Would you look in the pocket of my coat and bring it over?"

Chris returned card in hand, "This is for you. It's from all of us."

"Open it now?" They nodded. As I separated card from envelope a photo slipped out onto my dress.

I looked it. Then, I looked at Chris, Jason, and Neil. "It's you! It's *all* of you!" It was a photo of my group in 1988. They were standing so close together that each man's body touched the next. They looked healthy, vibrant, beautiful, perfectly perfect. A photo of all the men I interviewed in the fall of 1988 for an AIDS group I was to lead.

Neil said quietly, "I don't remember who took the photo. Maybe it was Vito because he's not in it."

Jason motioned to his coat again. "Chris, I should have asked to bring all my stuff over here."

"Sure." Chris returned holding a coat and a cane. Jason's cane?

"When did this happen?" I asked.

"It's been a while now. I've just usually left it at the reception desk, but there's no need to hide it anymore. I didn't want a repeat of the hospital where they said I looked too symptomatic to lead a group."

Jason looked forlorn and shrunken on his folding chair. "Here, I'll show you." Wincing, he slowly pulled up his pant leg. "I have Elephantiasis."[29]

It was ghastly. Jason's leg was swollen to twice the size it should have been.

"Oh my god, Jason," was all I could say. His skin wasn't skin. It looked like the hide of an elephant. My stomach flipped.

"How long has this existed?" I was stunned. How is it possible this thin young handsome man has an obese, distorted leg. Jason grimaced in pain as he pulled his pant leg down. He leaned back on his folding chair, his eyes full of emotion. In a moment, he faced me and forced a smile. His eyes were drastically sad, his voice weak, his body covered in pain. "We should end the session."

No one moved for a few minutes, we couldn't. Finally, each of us stood up in our own way. Jason leaned on his cane and grimaced. Neil's KS was now visible, his pain no longer hidden under clothing. Chris was agile. There was no evidence of pain or AIDS. I wobbled on my wooden crutch attempting a vertical position.

For many reasons, none of us were doing a decent job standing up. Once again, I failed to navigate my swing coat as it entwined with crutches. Chris grasped my arm to steady me, then whispered, "Can I stay in touch with you? Would you mind if we met or if I called once a month?"

"Absolutely! I'd love that. It'd be great to see you, whenever you want." My crutch tilted. Both Chris and Neil steadied me.

We just stood there. The four of us.

"I don't want to let go," Neil confessed.

"Good, because I'll fall over."

Neil kept holding my arm, then turned to hug me. Jason and Chris joined us. We hugged for a long time. No one moved.

"How do we leave if we keep doing this?" Neil laughed.

With perfect timing, Chris announced, "Let's stay like this. Like in the last episode of Mary Tylor Moore's TV show. You guys remember the scene where they couldn't stop hugging, so they moved as a unit and shuffled out the door still hugging each other."

"Chris." I lamented, "Plaster doesn't shuffle. We'll just have to stay this way."

"I can't shuffle, either. We have to stay put," Jason winced.

Then, once again the janitor's buckets rattled, "Hey, you guys done in here?"

"Yes." A quartet replied, loudly trumpeting the janitor's bucket banging. Slowly we un-hugged, limped, and grimaced to the doorway. We kept bumping into each other trying to mauver down the narrow hallway. Somehow, we reached the lobby. I waved to the empty reception desk with a last goodbye to the memory of Long Eyelashes.

Once outside, we stood there. I don't know how long we stood there. We wanted to capture time and hold it hostage.

Finally, someone said, "I'm going this way."

"You need help getting a taxi?" Chris asked.

"I'm fine."

Jason winced, "I need to get home. My leg hurts."

Neil took charge. "Let's get him home."

Chris, Neil, and Jason turned west. I turned east.

"Should I watch them walk away? Or should I close my eyes and forever hold their image between my eyelids?" I just stood there shivering from the cold wind. That's not true. It wasn't the wind making me shiver.

Chapter 37
Time

A few days later, Chris called. I heard his voice collapse, then, "Jason died yesterday."

"What!"

"When we were walking him home, he said he wasn't going to die until the group was finished. No matter what, he was going to keep his pledge." I was in shock. Chris broke the silence, "Can I come to your office later this month?"

A few weeks later, there he was. "I've got some good news. Vito is in town, doing multitudes of things, of course." Chris sighed, then looked away, "The bad news is, Neil passed last week."

Jason, Neil, Richard, Thomas, Matthew, Fernando, and my mother.

"I'll come visit the first Wednesday of each month at 5:00."

"Wonderful."

Chris came to my office the first Wednesday of each month until September 1990.

Confession: I have been writing this memory nearly thirty years and for thirty years my men have been in my head, clear as day. Eight handsome young men seated in a circle enthusiastically talking about what they did during the week and excited about what they planned for next week. During the life of the group, I unconsciously built an impregnable wall of denial only letting me see healthy men until the last few months.

Chapter 38
A Promise to Not Die

In the end, I kept my promise to the GMHC administrator. I have written about the group, and I ran the group solo. My advice about solo leading a group therapy: Never do that.

When I began working with my group, I quickly realized their emotional vulnerability required mine. They had no time to waste, and I had to keep up. I had to shift my philosophical perspective to an analytic theory that was coming of age in the 1980s. This theory prized the power of relationships, authenticity, and mutuality. However, making a shift from one theoretical perspective to another is about as easy as learning Sanskrit in a windstorm.

As I mentioned, it wasn't until the second year that their symptoms aggressively manifested, and their deaths slowly began. I not prepared. The only preparation I could muster was denial.

Initially, writing about my men felt exciting. Each chapter gave each man breath. This continued until I began writing about their deaths. These later chapters left me tearful with little desire to write the next. I often closed the computer, looked at their photo and 'forgot' I was writing this book, which is why it has taken thirty-years to complete. Yet, within those thirty years I built my private practice and did quite well professionally. In 2008, I moved to Arizona to marry. Now, my private practice is in Sedona, Arizona. Many of my New York City patients have remained with me, online.

Vito was the only member to outlive everyone in the group. The last time I saw him, I was Christmas shopping, December 1990. As I was walking down Fifth Avenue, I saw him. I saw Vito's pink cap. At the time, I didn't know Vito died November 1990, a month earlier.

Only after he was gone, only after they were all gone, did the pink cap morph into an unattainable faint image darting in and out of my periphery.

Notes

[1] Vito Russo, historian, lecturer, and author of *The Celluloid Closet: Homosexuality in the Movies* (1981, New York, Harper & Row). Russo was a Founding Member of the Gay and Lesbian Alliance Against Defamation (GLAAD), and an organizer of Gay Activists Alliance (GAA). The latter was a social organization that held Movie Nights led by Russo. This experience influenced his writing about gays in film. He also produced and co-hosted a public access series called *Our Time* that focused on gay culture, politics, and news. Russo became the National Publicity Director for the 1985 Oscar-winning documentary film *The Times of Harvey Milk*. Russo's involvement led to awards from the International Gay and Lesbian Film Festival and the Human Rights Campaign Fund. Russo's book *The Celluloid Closet: Homosexuality in the Movies* became a documentary in 1996 within which Russo was the focus. He was also a storyteller in *Common Threads: Stories from the Quilt* (1989), a documentary about the *Names Project AIDS Memorial Quilt*. Russo was the main focal point of the documentaries, *Vito* (2011), *Outspoken: A Vito Russo Reader – Reel One* (2012), *Reel Two* (2012). Michael Sciavi wrote the book, *Celluloid Activist: The Life and Times of Vito Russo* (2011). Lastly, Russo was co-author of *Voices from the Front* (published posthumously, 2001). All these

achievements paled compared to Vito's tenderness and generosity.

[2] Acquired Immunodeficiency Syndrome (AIDS). A chronic usually life-threatening condition stemming from Human Immunodeficiency Virus (HIV). HIV effects the body's immune system leaving it victim to infection and disease.

[3] Gay Men's Health Crisis (GMHC). Founded in 1982. Founders: Nathan Fain, Larry Kramer, Lawrence D. Mass, Paul Popham, Paul Rapoport and Edmund White. In the 1980s, it was the largest volunteer AIDS organization in the world. Organized for the prevention, support, and advocacy related to AIDS and HIV.

[4] Carlos Castaneda, *Journey to Ixtlan: The Lessons of Don Juan*. (New York: Washington Square Press, 1972), 40.

[5] Franz Kafka, *The Zürau Aphorisms (1917–1918)*. Kafka's notebook published posthumously, (Germany: Kiepenheuer & Witsch, 1931). A collection of Kafka's philosophical, metaphysical musings written on slips of paper while visiting his sister to recuperate from tuberculosis. Kafka suffered from stress-related illnesses creating depressive moods and intense anxiety, both would have psychologically influenced his thinking about the mind, his level of emotional suffering, as well as his existence within the Self and within nature. *The Zürau Aphorisms* was originally titled, *Betrachtungen über Sünde, Hoffnung, Leid und den wahren Weg (Reflections on Sin, Hope, Suffering, and the True Way*, 1931). Franz Kafka, *Aphorisms*, translated by Willa and Edwin Muir and Michael Hofmann, New York: Schocken Books/Penguin/Random House, 2015), 7.

[6] Saint Vitus dance or Sydenham's Chorea. A disorder that led to the Salem witch trials in Massachusetts between 1692 and 1693. Symptoms were uncontrollable manic movements, slurred speech, rapid involuntary twitching involving all parts of the body and face. These movements were an indication of witchery and

bewitching used during the witch trials. However, the real ontology of Saint Vitus dance disorder arose from eating ergot-tainted rye.

[7] Apollonius of Rhodes, *Argonautica*, (Greece, 3rd century BC). The only existing ancient Hellenistic epic poem. The *Argonautica* tells the mythic voyage of Jason, blood-line descendant to the throne, who was sent away by his uncle, the latter having usurped succession to the throne rightly due Jason's father. The king/uncle feared losing his position to Jason and decided to rid himself of Jason's presence/threat to the throne. In the meantime, the king/uncle had received many oracle warning as well as visitation from haunting ghosts, all of whom say he shouldn't have taken the throne. So, the king swears/promises to give the throne to Jason if he voyages to and returns home with the Golden Fleece (which was initially Jason's idea because the Queen of the Greek gods, Hera, put words in Jason's mouth for many reasons related to the King of the gods, Zeus' philandering). Jason's uncle, who fears the gods, a normal reaction at the time, says he'll actually give up the throne to Jason if he sails to Colchis, a difficult to reach location, and if Jason retrieves the Golden Fleece, guarded by a dragon with severe insomnia, thus making it truly difficult to fetch the fleece due to the possibility of being eaten by the dragon. Obviously, this is a potentially lousy life-threatening journey and Jason needs back-up, so he enlists a bunch of heroes, such as Hercules and forty-nine other herculean-types to go with him on a ship named Argo, hence the heroes are called Argonauts. But, one of the heroes is left behind, a woman named Atalanta because she's not like the men and shouldn't have the power of being with the men and especially she shouldn't be the leader amongst a group of guys (because she doesn't have AIDS and is odd man out, then). There are many variations of this story, so don't quote me.

[8] *Everyman*. A morality play written by Peter Dorland, produced in Britain in 1901. The story is taken from a late 15th century morality play, *The Summoning of Everyman*, author unknown. The only part of the play I like is that Everyman tries to convince men to accompany him to mutually improve each other's life, i.e., Jason's insistence that together, every man in my group pledged to not die and remain with each other for emotional support. I'm not thrilled with the other messages in the play, it's just this one particular message. Don't apply any other meaning, because it's just this one message out of the entire play that works here.

[9] Thomas De Quincy, *Confessions of an English Opium Eater, London Magazine,* (First publication: London, 1823). (Revised edition: Barry Milligan, ed. Penguin Classics, 2003), 7.

[10] Popul Today, "AIDS Worldwide," R. Yared, 1989, February: 17 (2):4.

[11] ACT UP, acronym for AIDS Coalition to Unleash Power. An activist political group rallying/working to end the AIDS pandemic and increase societal AIDS awareness through activism.

[12] Nietzsche, Friedrich. *The Gay Science* (1882). Book in which Nietzsche proclaimed the death of God. Also titled, *The Joyful Wisdom*. Walter Kaufmann, translator, (New York: Vintage Books, 1974).

[13] James Kirkwood and Nicholas Dante, playwriters, *A Chorus Line.* "One," a song from the original score of the 1975 Broadway musical. Music by Marvin Hamlisch; lyrics, Edward Kleban. 1976 Tony Award for Best Musical, Best Book of a Musical, Best Original Score. Pulitzer Prize for Drama, Olivier Award for Best Musical.

[14] Olive Higgins Prouty's book, *Now, Voyager,* (1941). Film, *Now Voyager* (Hollywood: 1942), starring Bette Davis, Paul Henreid and Claude Rains. Directed by Irving Rapper. Screenplay by

Casey Robinson. Exact quote from film: "Oh, Jerry, don't let's ask for the moon. We have the stars."

[15] Video Transcript of "Why We Fight," speech by Vito Russo at the ACT UP Demonstration in Albany, NY, May 9, 1988 and the ACT UP Demonstration at the Department of Health and Human Services, Washington D.C. October 10, 1988. https://actupny.org/documents/whfight.html

[16] Gustav Vigeland's Sculpture garden in Frogner Park, Oslo, Norway was mostly completed in 1919. Vigeland was also the designer of the Nobel Peace Prize medal.

[17] *Common Threads: Stories from the Quilt (1989)*. Documentary about the *Names Project AIDS Memorial Quilt*. Vito Russo is one of the storytellers in the documentary. He talks about his partner, Jeffrey Sevcik who died from AIDS at age 30. Documentary written by Rob Epstein, Jeffrey Friedman, Cindy Ruskin. *Common Threads* won the Academy Award for Best Documentary Feature in 1990, as well as the Interfilm Award at the 1990 Berlin Film Festival, a GLAAD Media Award for Best TV Documentary, and a Peabody Award.

[18] Charles Dickens, *The Haunted House,* Published in *All the Year Round, (Extra Christmas Edition,* Volume 13, 1859). A story about ghosts who are not really ghosts or 'not yet ghosts.' Dickens' story was meant/written as metaphor for sorrow, prejudice, and fear.

[19] Vito Russo, "Why We Fight" speech (video transcript) at Washington DC, *ACT UP Seize Control of FDA Protest*, October 10, 1988. Same rally/speech previously held in Albany, NY, May 9, 1988.

http://actupny.org/documents/whfighthtml

[20] Initially, AZT was typically prescribed at 400 mg every four hours, day and night. "The paucity of alternatives for treating HIV/AIDS at that time unambiguously affirmed the health

risk/benefit ratio, with inevitable slow, disfiguring, and painful death from HIV outweighing the drug's side-effect of transient anemia and malaise."

https://en.wikipedia.org/wiki/Zidovudine

[21] Celia Farber, "Sins of Omission: AIDS and the AZT Scandal," (New York: *SPIN Magazine,* November 1989), "According to the 8/17/89 government announcement, '3,200 early ARC AIDS Related Complex (ARC, a now-obsolete medical term for pre-AIDS illness) and asymptomatic patients were divided into two groups, one given AZT and one placebo, and followed for two years. The two groups were distinguished by T-4 cell counts; one group had less than 500, the other more than 500. These two were then divided into three groups each: high-dose AZT, low-dose AZT, and placebo. In the group with more than 500 T-4 cells, AZT had no effect. In the other group, it was concluded that low-dose AZT was the most effective, followed by high-dose. All in all, 36 out of 900 developed AIDS in the two AZT groups combined, and 38 out of 450 in the placebo group. 'HIV-positive [individuals] are twice as likely to get AIDS if they don't take AZT.'"

"During the 1980s, most people with AIDS died from opportunistic infections, especially Pneumocystic Carinii Pneumonia (PCP) and Kaposi's Sarcoma (KS). These infections took lives before the AIDS virus did. AZT worked in such a way that PCP and KS increased rather than decreased. After an initial boost in T-4 cell count, AZT crippled and soon, actually blocked T-4 cells, white blood cells, the immune system cells, the cells engaged to help guard the body against a multitude of infectious diseases. As a result, many HIV infected people died from AZT poisoning, not AIDS. KS and PCP were both treatable diseases in the 1980s. Treatable with meds like Aerosolized Pentamidine that might have extended life or at least, slowed down the AIDS virus."

[22] Michael Byrne, "A Brief History of AZT, HIV's First 'Ray of Hope,'" (*Vice*, 2015) https://www.vice.com/en/article/mgb48x/happy-birthday-to-azt-the-first-effective-hiv-treatment.

[23] Y.P. Mingle & S.K. Sharm, eds., *API Textbook of Medicine*, 9th ed., 2 Vol set, 1st edition, 1969, (India: Jaypee Brothers Medical Publisher, Ltd, 2012), 1032.

"Opportunistic Infections (OIs) is a disease caused by microbial agents(s) in hosts with defects in humoral and cell mediated immunity-immuno-compromise secondary to human immunodeficiency virus (HIV) infection, use of immunomodulatory agents (including steroids and anticancer drugs) were emerging as predisposing factors to OIs. Opportunistic infections (OIs) may serve as indicators of underlying HIV infection.

Mortality among HIV-infected individuals is due to improper awareness and consequent poor clinical management of OIs. HIV load increases in the presence of ongoing OIs, thus accelerating progression to clinical acquired immunodeficiency syndrome (AIDS).

Changes in the C4 lymphocyte count occur with the institution of highly active antiretroviral therapy (HAART) which in turn results in changes in OIs epidemiology, clinical presentation and treatment outcomes. As HAART results in reconstitution of the immune system – certain OIs respond to HAART alone. However, the ensuing immune medicated inflammatory response may present as a paradoxical worsening of disease. It is therefore essential to be able to recognize and treat OIs prior to the institution of antiretroviral agents. OIs plays a role in the clinical staging of HIV infection. OIs may present as indolent chronic infections (pyrexia of unknown origin), reactivation of latent infections, or as acute medical emergencies. They may affect single or multiple organ systems."

[24] Joseph Sonnabend, MD, "Remembering the Original AZT Trial, *(POZ,* 2011) https://www.poz.com/blog/-v-behaviorurldefaul

[25] Reuters, "Growing Benefit Seen in AIDS Drug," *New York Times*, 1988. https://timesmachine.nytimes.com/timesmachine/1988/05/14/073988.html

Marlene Cimons, "AZT Found to Delay AIDS in Those Free of Symptoms," *Los Angeles Times*, 1989. https://www.latimes.com/archives/la-xpm-1989-08-18-mn-561-story.html

[26] *The Who*, a rock group that produced the album, *Tommy*. One song is about a Pinball World Championship won by a deaf, dumb, and blind kid who becomes the Pinball Wizard, metaphor for the struggles, betrayals and denials suffered by Jesus. (US: Decca, UK: Track Records), 1969.

[27] John Lauritsen, "First Things First: Some Thoughts on the 'AIDS Virus' and AZT," *New York Native,* 1987, 1, 14–16.https://publishing.cdlib.org/ucpressebooks/view?docId=ft1s20045x&chunk.id=d0e7714&toc.id=d0e7560&brand=ucPress.

[28] John Lauritsen, "Incompetency in AIDS Epidemiology," *Forum on Causes of AIDS*, New York: 1988).

[29] Ananya Mandal, MD, "Elephantiasis refers to a parasitic infection that causes extreme swelling in the arms and legs. The disease is caused by the filarial worm, which is transmitted from human to human via the female mosquito when it takes a blood meal. The parasite grows into an adult worm that lives in the lymphatic system of humans." (https://www.news-medical.not, 2014).

www.ingramcontent.com/pod-product-compliance
Lightning Source LLC
Chambersburg PA
CBHW070628220526
45466CB00001B/120